TINTNER

HEAD INJURY

Volume 10 in the Series

Major Problems in Neurology

SIR JOHN WALTON, TD, MD, DSc, FRCP
Consulting Editor

OTHER MONOGRAPHS IN THE SERIES

PUBLISHED

Barnett, Foster and Hudgson: **Syringomyelia,** *1973*
Dubowitz and Brooke: **Muscle Biopsy: A Modern Approach,** *1973*
Pallis and Lewis: **The Neurology of Gastrointestinal Disease,** *1974*
Hutchinson and Acheson: **Strokes,** *1975*
Gubbay: **The Clumsy Child,** *1975*
Hankinson and Banna: **Pituitary and Parapituitary Tumours,** *1976*
Donaldson: **Neurology of Pregnancy,** *1977*
Behan and Currie: **Clinical Neuroimmunology,** *1978*
Harper: **Myotonic Dystrophy,** *1979*

Head Injury

N. E. F. CARTLIDGE, MB, BS, FRCP

Senior Lecturer in Neurology, University of Newcastle upon Tyne;
Consultant Neurologist, Newcastle Area Health Authority (Teaching),
and Honorary Consultant Neurologist, Northern Regional Health Authority.

D. A. SHAW, MB, ChB, FRCP, FRCP(Edin.)

Professor of Clinical Neurology, University of Newcastle upon Tyne;
Honorary Consultant Neurologist, Newcastle Area Health Authority (Teaching)
and Northern Regional Health Authority.

With a contribution by

R. M. KALBAG, MSc, MB, BS, FRCS
Consultant Neurosurgeon, Regional Neurological Centre, Newcastle General
Hospital.

1981

W. B. Saunders Company Ltd   London · Philadelphia · Toronto

W. B. Saunders Company Ltd: 1 St Anne's Road
Eastbourne, East Sussex BN21 3UN

West Washington Square
Philadelphia, PA 19105

1 Goldthorne Avenue
Toronto, Ontario M8Z 5T9

British Library Cataloguing in Publication Data

Cartlidge, N. E. F.
    Head injury.
    1. Head — Wounds and injuries
    I. Title   II. Shaw, D.
    617'.51   RD521

Head Injury

ISBN 0-7216-2443-X

Printed at The Lavenham Press Ltd, Lavenham, Suffolk, England.

Print Number: 9 8 7 6 5 4 3 2 1

Foreword

While injuries to the head, and especially those resulting from warfare, have occupied the time and interest of physicians and surgeons for many centuries the startling increases in industrial injury which followed the Industrial Revolution and the many accidental injuries resulting from the advent of mechanical methods of transport have meant that increasing attention has been focused upon this problem. In civil life, road accidents are an increasingly important cause of serious head injury despite widespread publicity and legislation relating to the wearing of protective helmets (for motorcyclists) and seat-belts (for car drivers) and despite the introduction of many measures aimed at accident prevention. Hence the consequential mortality and morbidity mean that head injury is a major scourge of modern society which has therefore received a great deal of well-deserved attention in the medical literature. However, most such writings have come from the neurosurgeons, upon whose shoulders the major burden of caring for these patients has fallen. This monograph, written by two neurologists, attempts a somewhat different approach, although a useful succinct chapter on management including a summary of surgical techniques written by their colleague Mr R. M. Kalbag fittingly concludes the volume.

What the authors have done is to review comprehensively the relevant literature on this topic and to analyse in detail their personal findings based upon a detailed examination and follow-up study of 425 consecutive and unselected patients with head injury admitted to a neurosurgical unit in Newcastle upon Tyne over the course of 21 months.

As all of the patients were examined according to a standard protocol by one of the authors, who was also responsible for detailed assessment of the sequelae, both organic and psychiatric, which were observed on follow-up examination, considerable consistency in assessment was achieved, a feature which makes this survey particularly valuable.

It would be inappropriate in a foreword such as this to highlight the detailed findings and conclusions of the study, as readers of this well-written and succinct survey will wish to judge and consider these for themselves. There were a few surprises; thus, in a series containing many severely injured patients there were only two cases of severe post-traumatic dementia. However, the information which the authors give upon epidemiology, medical and social consequences, the assessment of coma and of neurological findings and their significance, upon post-traumatic headache and dizziness, the postconcussional syndrome, and upon medical, neurological and psychiatric sequelae will in my view make this volume required reading for all neurologists, anaesthetists, neurosurgeons, otolaryngologists, psychiatrists and others who are concerned with head injury and its sequelae in all aspects. Even lawyers concerned with the medicolegal implications of head injury could profit from reading many parts of it. I have found it both readable and informative.

Newcastle upon Tyne, 1981   John N. Walton

Preface

Head injury and its consequences cast a blight on the health statistics of most nations and a shadow on the lives of countless individuals and families. The present sad state of affairs is unlikely to improve without sustained effort in many different fields — industrial, mechanical and sociological, as well as medical. It seems that evidence supporting measures to reduce the accident toll must be overwhelming before even tardy legislative response can be expected.

The study of head injury, on which this book is based, was undertaken with two main questions in mind. The first related to the postconcussional syndrome and the possibility that detailed enquiry about antecedent factors of divers kinds might lead to a better understanding of its nature. The second concerned accidents themselves, as opposed to their medical consequences, in the hope that an epidemiological approach to them might yield clues as to possible methods of prevention beyond those already identified. Inevitably the study moved in directions other than those primarily intended and the original aims were not completely fulfilled. We collected many data which eventually proved to be superfluous and omitted others which might have been valuable. The study, like so many others, raised questions that it had not anticipated. Nevertheless we were able to reach some conclusions about the sequelae of head injury and they are presented in these pages.

The suggestion that the results of the study might be incorporated in a monograph was made by Sir John Walton and gratefully accepted. We have attempted to weave the Newcastle experience into a broader review of the subject and to match it against the results of other studies. In our task we have been helped immeasurably by Sir John's advice, encouragement and forbearance and we have been grateful for his expert editorship.

Several people other than ourselves made major contributions to the study. Mr Ram Kalbag, the Consultant Neurosurgeon under whose care all the patients were admitted to the Regional Neurological Centre, gave willing help and advice based on vast experience, and he wrote the final chapter of the book. Dr Ken Davison, Consultant Psychiatrist at the Newcastle General Hospital, gave invaluable help in the original design of the study, advised on its psychiatric aspects and saw all the patients with major psychiatric problems. Dr Alan Craft participated willingly in some follow-up clinics and Miss Pat Longley, of the Department of Clinical Neurophysiology at the Regional Neurological Centre, gave facilities and expert help in making the electronystagmographic recordings. Miss Judith Partridge, the social worker appointed to the study, made a major contribution in its design and in the original and follow-up social assessments. The smooth running of the study was largely due to her, to her successor Mrs Y. Peterson and to several secretaries within the department who gave willing administrative assistance. For the preparation of manuscripts we are greatly indebted to Mrs Mavis Ferguson, Miss Susan Alcock and Mrs Anita Kay.

The Newcastle Regional Hospital Board, later to become the Northern Regional Health Authority in the reorganized National Health Service, generously financed and supported the study. It made available to us the resources of its statistical department to whose head, Mr Angus McNay, we are indebted for much help and advice. Members of his staff, particularly Miss Shirley Smolt, gave invaluable assistance with the computer analyses.

Appropriate and grateful acknowledgements appear with some of the illustrations but we would thank Dr Alan Craft for Figures 3.1 and 3.2, Dr N. I. Chalat and the Laryngoscope Company for Figure 3.3 and Dr J. B. Foster for Figure 3.4. The Department of Transport and the Controller, Her Majesty's Stationery Office, kindly allowed us to publish Figure 4.1 and Table 4.1.

Finally, it is a pleasure to acknowledge all the help that we received from the publishers, W. B. Saunders Company Ltd.

Newcastle upon Tyne   N. E. F. Cartlidge
1981   D. A. Shaw

Contents

To the memory
of
HENRY MILLER

CHAPTER ONE

Introduction

Head injury is a subject that features prominently in early medical writings. There is a reference to 'instructions concerning a gaping wound in the head, penetrating to the bone, smashing the skull, rending open the brain . . . ' in what has come to be known as the Edwin Smith Papyrus, the oldest known medical text (Figure 1.1).

Edwin Smith was born in Connecticut in 1822 but lived for many years in Egypt. In 1862 he purchased from an Egyptian merchant in Thebes a papyrus containing twenty-one and a half columns of legend. Some time after his death, Edwin Smith's daughter gave the papyrus to the New York Historical Society where it lay untouched for many years. Eventually it was discovered by a scholar from the University of Chicago called Breasted, who translated and published it (Breasted, 1930). The papyrus is thought to have originated in the fourth dynasty of the old kingdom of Egypt and is thus estimated to be approximately 4 500 years old.

The Edwin Smith Papyrus contains descriptions of 48 cases of bodily trauma amongst which there were 27 head injuries; the passage quoted above refers to one of these. It thus provides a fitting introduction to the present volume, which addresses itself to the same problem whilst humbly recognizing that it is unlikely to achieve quite the same permanence.

Statistical figures on accidental injury, whatever their source, are appalling. In most advanced countries today, accident comes fourth in order of frequency as a cause of death. Only ischaemic heart disease, cancer and cerebrovascular disease are higher on the list. Even more striking perhaps is the fact that during the first four decades of life accident is the single most common cause of death. It is remarkable that societies which are capable of great compassion and generosity towards small numbers of individuals afflicted by rare diseases, and which can be genuinely affected by news of sudden disaster costing a handful of lives, can at the same time accept with apparent equanimity an outrageous toll of dead and maimed as a result of domestic, industrial and traffic accidents, many of which are preventable. It is one of the less attractive features of modern civilization that it lacks the social conscience and the political will to set a higher price on the safety and well-being of its individual members.

Accident statistics are available from a number of different countries. In the United States, it is estimated that there are as many as 50 million accidental injuries of one sort or another each year involving one in four of the total population (Feiring and Brock, 1974). As a result of these accidents, 44 million people receive medical attention, 2 million require hospital care and over 100 000 die. In Canada, trauma is the principal cause of death between the ages of two and 44 years (Hay, 1967); for all ages, accident is the third most common cause of death (Traffic Injury Research Foundation of Canada, 1972). Approximately half a million patients are admitted annually to hospitals in England and Wales because of accidents and 18 000 of them die (HIPE, 1976). The injury figures in Scotland are similar (SHIPS, 1975) and in one major hospital in Glasgow it has been estimated that trauma accounts for over one-third of all acute surgical admissions (Patel, 1977).

In all of these accidents, fatal or otherwise, the commonest single site of injury is the head. Of the 50 million accidental injuries that occur annually in the United States, 3 million are head injuries. Analysis of the England and Wales figures shows that 20 per cent of those admitted to hospital as a result of trauma have suffered a head injury and the annual total amounts to more than 100 000. In Scotland, with a population of 5 million, 15 000 patients with head injury are admitted to hospital each year. The mortality figures for head injury are even more devastating. Of those who die as a result of accidents, no less than 70 per cent do so because of their head injuries (Gogler, 1965; NINCDS, 1976).

The cost of all these accidents and injuries in terms of human suffering is immeasurable. Although of secondary importance, there is also a financial cost and various attempts have been made, admittedly speculative in some instances, to estimate the economic implications. The National Institute of Neurological and Communicative

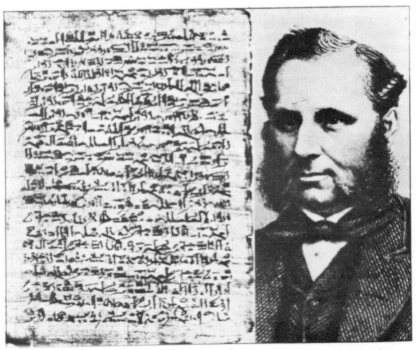

Figure 1.1.   Edwin Smith and an extract from the Papyrus.

Disorders and Stroke has assessed the annual cost of care for patients with head injuries in the United States of America at 3 billion dollars. The figure includes a calculation of 1000 dollars a year for each patient for medical fees, speech therapy, special education and other expenses (NINCDS, 1976). It compares with a cost of 2 billion dollars a year for patients with epilepsy and 12.5 billion dollars a year for stroke cases. The calculation does not, however, take any account of the economic cost to the community in terms of lost earnings, which has been estimated at 100 billion dollars per decade (Haddon, 1971). Scaled down appropriately for the different population size, the economic costs in the United Kingdom are much the same as they are in the United States. As far back as 1963 it was estimated that the total annual cost to the nation of all accidents was around 500 million pounds (Beckingsale, 1963). Road accidents alone in 1970 were estimated to cost the nation 1 million pounds a day (Road Accidents, 1972); this had risen to almost 2 million pounds a day by 1974 (Road Accidents Great Britain, 1976). These figures indicate that the total cost of all accidents in the United Kingdom must be enormous.

Whilst these crude statistics give us an idea of the magnitude of the accident and head injury problem in broad terms, there is not a great deal of detailed epidemiological information derived from community studies. Rune (1970) carried out a cumulative prevalence survey of head injury in children aged seven to 16 years in the Swedish provincial town of Umeå. Parents were asked if their children had ever suffered a blow to the head of sufficient severity to cause them serious worry. The survey covered 5105 children; 15 per cent of them had had at least one such injury. Table 1.1 shows the percentage risk of head injury in children in a year as calculated by Rune. This study had the limitations of all retrospective surveys, but it does give an indication of the size of the hazard and it confirms that head injury is of common occurrence in the young.

Table 1.1. Percentage risk of children suffering head injury in one year by age and sex (M = male, F = female) — Umeå 1967.

	1 yr		1-3 yrs		4-6 yrs		7-9 yrs		10-16 yrs	
	M	F	M	F	M	F	M	F	M	F
Head Injury	0.9	0.9	1.7	1.4	1.7	1.2	1.6	0.8	1.6	0.8
Concussion	0.6	0.5	0.9	0.8	1.0	0.7	1.1	0.6	1.0	0.6
Unconsciousness	0.2	0.2	0.5	0.5	0.5	0.4	0.7	0.4	0.7	0.4

The National Study of General Practice, carried out in 1970/71 in England and Wales, provided some statistics on general practitioner consultations including information on the incidence of head injury. Table 1.2 is based on this study and shows the patient consulting rates per thousand of population per year for head injury (Field, 1976). If these figures are representative of the United Kingdom as a whole, the number of people consulting a general practitioner because of head injury in the course of a year is of the order of 45 000 males and 23 000 females.

Table 1.2. Patients consulting general practitioners for head injury in England and Wales 1970-71. Rates per 1000 population.

	All ages	0—	5—	15	25	45	65	75 & over
Males	1.9	2.2	1.9	3.9	1.5	1.1	1.1	1.6
Females	0.9	1.9	1.1	1.2	0.6	0.5	0.5	1.1

Little information is available about the number of patients with head injury who attend emergency departments but do not need to be admitted to hospital. A paediatric study in Canada (Klonoff, 1971) produced evidence that at least as many children with head injury were discharged after being seen in a casualty department as were admitted. Until recently, no such information was available as regards adults. However, the Scottish Head Injury Management Study (SHIMS, 1977) was designed to look particularly at this problem. The study has shown that head injuries account for 10 per cent of all new attendances at accident and emergency departments in Scotland; extrapolation from the figures collected in the two-week sample period indicates that there are approximately 84 000 head injury attendances in casualty departments in Scottish hospitals per annum. The figure for the United Kingdom as a whole is approximately 1 million. Twenty-two per cent of the patients in the study sample were admitted to hospital and the remainder were discharged. The survey thus confirms the suggestion, made previously by Jennett (1975), that only a quarter to a fifth of people attending casualty departments after head injury are actually admitted to hospital.

Information about those head injuries that do not lead to hospital admission is somewhat scanty. Obviously the policy regarding admission will vary from hospital to hospital but it is certainly true that there may be persisting symptoms, even resulting in loss of work and permanent disability, in patients whose initial injury is not thought worthy of hospitalization. Out-patient experience teaches us that a number of patients continue to complain of symptoms following head injuries for which they never sought medical advice at the time.

Most of the detailed statistical information available on head injuries comes from hospital studies. In the United Kingdom an annual report is published by Her Majesty's Stationery Office called the Hospital In-patient Enquiry. This gives detailed information on categories of illness and patterns of admission and discharge of National Health Service patients in all hospitals in England and Wales. Table 1.3 is taken from the Hospital In-patient Enquiry of 1972 and shows the hospital discharges

Table 1.3.   Hospital discharge for head injury, England and Wales, 1972.

Age	Males	Females	Total
0—4	11 390	8 002	19 392
5—14	23 017	11 502	34 519
15—19	13 433	4 922	18 355
20—24	11 835	3 314	15 149
25—34	11 624	3 610	15 234
35—44	6 518	2 936	9 454
45—64	11 263	5 905	17 168
65—74	3 447	3 124	6 571
75 and over	2 083	4 091	6 174
Totals all ages	*94 610*	*47 406*	*142 016*

under the category of head injury for that year. Males outnumber females by almost two to one and more than half of those who had been in hospital were under the age of 20. When the figures are adjusted for the age and sex structure of the population as a whole, it is quite apparent that males at all ages are at an increased risk of admission to hospital as a result of head injury, although the differences at the extremes of life are marginal. A number of independent studies have confirmed the Hospital In-patient Enquiry statistics showing the predominance of head injuries in males and in the younger age groups. In children, Burkinshaw (1960) and Partington (1960) both showed at least a 2 to 1 male predominance in figures for hospital admission following head injury. The peak incidence was between the ages of six and 10 years. A more recent prospective study of 200 childhood head injuries in Newcastle gave comparable figures, which are illustrated in Table 1.4 (Craft, Shaw and Cartlidge, 1972).

Reports from various parts of the world on hospital surveys of head injuries in adults give fairly consistent findings. Rowbotham et al (1954) reported on 1000 adult patients admitted to hospital with head injury: a high proportion were in the younger age groups and the male/female ratio was four to one. Ten years later Barr and Ralston (1964) reported very similar findings. Steadman and Graham (1970) reviewed a series of 404 head-injured patients in Cardiff who required hospitalization. There was a high proportion of patients in the 10 to 25 years age bracket. In the whole series, the number of males exceeded that of females by 2.5 to one. Kerr, Kay and Lassman (1971), again from Newcastle, confirmed a male preponderance in those with head injuries and,

Table 1.4. Age and sex distribution in 200 paediatric head injuries. From Craft, Shaw and Cartlidge (1972).

Age	<1	1	2	3	4	5	6	7	8	9	10	11	12	13	14
Male	10	14	7	9	9	7	16	13	11	6	10	9	5	3	2
Female	5	11	10	3	3	13	5	2	1	3	3	2	7	0	1
Total	15	25	17	12	12	20	21	15	12	9	13	11	12	3	3

as in the Cardiff study, they found in their series an excessive representation of patients in the younger age groups. Also, there was a male/female ratio of four to one. These British studies thus show consistency over a period of almost 20 years and very similar figures have emerged from research in many other parts of the world: Gurdjian and Thomas (1966) and Barber and Webster (1974) in the United States, Klonoff and Thompson (1969) and Hendrick, Harwood-Nash and Hudson (1964) in Canada, Kalyanaran (1974) in India, Selecki, Hoy and Ness (1967) in Australia, Chien (1970) in Taiwan, and Basauri and Rocamora (1968) in Chile. The age and sex distribution of head injury in these studies generally resembles that published in the United Kingdom series; there is wide confirmation of the enormous impact of head injuries on the whole population, and especially on the young and the males of the species.

There is thus ample evidence in national statistical reports and in the world medical literature as to the magnitude of the head injury problem and its appalling death toll. There is also a vast literature concerning the physical and psychological sequelae of head injury in those who survive; some of this will be reviewed in later chapters. Yet society seems reluctant to meet the challenge that these figures present. Might attitudes change with a more detailed knowledge of the many factors, both personal and environmental, that predispose to accidents? And might a deeper understanding of the factors that determine the outcome of head injury in those who survive facilitate their rehabilitation? With these questions in mind it was decided that a further study of the natural history of head injury was worth undertaking, and in the following chapters we present the results of a survey carried out in Newcastle in the years 1970 to 1971.

REFERENCES

Barber, J. & Webster, J. C. (1974) Head injuries — review of 150 cases. *Journal of the National Medical Association,* **66,** 201-204.
Barr, J. B. & Ralston, G. J. (1964) Head injuries in a peripheral hospital. *Lancet,* **ii,** 519-522.
Basauri, L. & Rocamora, R. J. (1968) Traumatismo encefalo cineano. *Neurocirugia,* **26,** 254-263.

Beckingsale, A. A. (1963) The cost of industrial accidents. *Royal Society of Arts,* London.

Breasted, J. H. (1930) *The Edwin Smith Surgical Papyrus.* Chicago: University of Chicago Press.

Burkinshaw, J. (1960) Head injuries in children. *Archives of Diseases of Childhood,* **35,** 205-214.

Chien, Y. C. (1970) Studies on the factors influencing the prognosis of head injuries based upon 1030 cases. *Journal of the Formosan Medical Association,* **69,** 22-35.

Craft, A. W., Shaw, D. A. & Cartlidge, N. E. F. (1972) Head injuries in children. *British Medical Journal,* **iv,** 200-203.

Feiring, E. H. & Brock, S. (1974) General considerations in injuries of the brain and spinal cord and their coverings. *Injuries of the Brain and Spinal Cord* (Ed.) Feiring, E. H. Chapter 1. New York: Springer Publishing.

Field, J. H. (1976) Epidemiology of head injuries in England and Wales. London: Her Majesty's Stationery Office.

Gogler, E. (1965) *Road Accidents.* Documenta Geigy Series Chirurgica, Geigy (U.K.).

Gurdjian, E. S. & Thomas, L. M. (1966) Management of head injury in the United States. *Head Injury* (Ed.) Caveness, W. F. & Walker, A. E. Philadelphia and Toronto: J. B. Lippincott.

Haddon, W. (1971) Logical framework for categorising highway safety phenomena and activity. *Journal of Trauma,* **11,** 65-69.

Hay, R. H. (1967) Neurosurgical aspects of traffic accidents: report of Sub-Committee of the Canadian Neurosurgical Society. *Canadian Medical Association Journal,* **97,** 1364-1368.

Hendrick, E. B., Harwood-Nash, D. C. F. & Hudson, A. R. (1964) Head injuries in children. *Clinical Neurosurgery,* **11,** 46-65.

HIPE (Hospital In-Patient Enquiry for the Year 1972) 1975. Department of Health and Social Security.

HIPE (Hospital In-Patient Enquiry for the Year 1973) 1976. Department of Health and Social Security.

Jennett, B. (1975) Who cares for head injuries? *British Medical Journal,* **iii,** 267-270.

Kalyanaran, S., Ramamurthi, B. & Ramamoorthy, K. (1974) An analysis of 2000 cases of head injury. *Neurology (India),* **18,** 3-11.

Kerr, T. A., Kay, D. W. & Lassman, L. P. (1971) Characteristics of patients, type of accident, and mortality in a consecutive series of head injuries admitted to a neurological unit. *British Journal of Preventive Medicine,* **25,** 179-185.

Klonoff, H. (1971) Head injuries in children — predisposing factors, accident conditions, accident proneness and sequelae. *American Journal of Public Health,* **61,** 2405-2417.

Klonoff, H. & Thompson, G. B. (1969) Epidemiology of head injuries in adults — a pilot study. *Canadian Medical Association Journal,* **100,** 235-241.

NINCDS (National Institute of Neurological and Communicative Disorders and Stroke) 1976.

Partington, M. W. (1960) The importance of accident proneness in the aetiology of head injuries in childhood. *Archives of Diseases of Childhood,* **35,** 215-223.

Patel, A. (1977) Problems for Accident and Emergency Departments. *Proceedings of a Symposium on Head Injuries held at the Royal College of Physicians and Surgeons, Glasgow.*

Road Accidents 1970 (in Great Britain) (1972) London: Her Majesty's Stationery Office.

Road Accidents Great Britain 1974 (1976) London: Her Majesty's Stationery Office.

Rowbotham, G. F., McIvor, I. N., Dicksson, J. & Bousfield, M. E. (1954) Analysis of 1400 cases of acute injury to the head. *British Medical Journal,* **i,** 726-729.

Rune, V. (1970) Acute head injuries in children. *Acta Paediatrica Scandinavica* (Supplement), **209.**

Selecki, B. R., Hoy, R. J. & Ness, P. (1967) A retrospective survey of neuro-traumatic admissions to a teaching hospital. Part I. General Aspects. *The Medical Journal of Australia,* **2,** 113-117.

SHIMS (Scottish Head Injury Management Study) 1977.

SHIPS (Scottish Hospital In-Patient Statistics 1974) 1975. Scottish Home and Health Department. Information Services Division of the Common Services Agency, Edinburgh.

Steadman, J. H. & Graham, J. G. (1970) Rehabilitation of the head injured. *Proceedings of the Royal Society of Medicine,* **63,** 23-26.

Traffic Injury Research Foundation of Canada (1972) Ottawa, Ontario, Canada.

CHAPTER TWO

The Newcastle Head Injury Study

Many important facts in medicine have been established on the basis of retrospective surveys, but there are inherent weaknesses in this method of study. The clinical data recorded for routine purposes are often unreliable and seldom are they adequate for the requirements of special study. There is also a serious risk of bias resulting from methods of selection and sampling. It is now generally accepted that, to be of maximum value, detailed study of any particular group of patients should be prospective so that the criteria for inclusion and the methods of data collection can be clearly defined beforehand.

In the case of head injury there have been a great many retrospective studies but remarkably few prospective ones. There are two of particular note which stand out as landmarks and which still form the basis of much of our traditional thinking about head injury. The first was that of Russell (1932). He examined 200 consecutive patients admitted to the surgical wards of the Edinburgh Royal Infirmary because of head injury, and the information that he collected laid the foundation of much of our present day knowledge of head injury. In particular he drew attention to the importance of post-traumatic amnesia. Some 10 years later a similar but more detailed study was undertaken in Boston under the direction of Denny-Brown (1945). He and his co-workers examined a total of 430 cases of head injury admitted to the Boston City Hospital, and recorded detailed information on the natural history of recovery in a selected group of 200. A number of important publications resulted from the Boston head injury survey and reference will be made to these in subsequent chapters. The study certainly provided some of the earliest information on post-traumatic headache and post-traumatic dizziness, and also on the psychiatric sequelae of head injury. Apart from these two major contributions, and the more recent studies of Jennett and his colleagues in Glasgow (Jennett et al, 1976), no other detailed prospective studies on unselected head injury patients seem to have been reported in the English literature.

The study on which this book is based concerns a group of patients admitted to a single neurosurgery unit over a period of 21 months and subsequently observed for at least two years. All were under the care of the same neurosurgeon (Mr. R. M. Kalbag)

7

and all were independently examined, both on admission to the study and at follow-up, by one of the authors (N.E.F.C.). In Newcastle there are two neurosurgical teams providing a regional head injury service; they share the workload on the basis of an alternate week duty system, so the patients included in the study comprised approximately half of the total admitted during the relevant period. The Newcastle General Hospital receives patients from a large geographical area (Figure 2.1). Newcastle itself has a population of only 250 000, but the head injury service caters for the needs of approximately a million people. The majority of patients with head injury requiring admission are brought directly to the hospital from the scene of the accident. Most come from the city of Newcastle itself or its near environs. A small proportion are transferred from other hospitals in the region, usually because of suspected intracranial bleeding. The admissions policy of the unit involved in the study is outlined in Chapter 13 which is concerned with management. For the purposes of our study, a patient was deemed to fall into the category of 'acute head injury' if the accident had occurred not more than 24 hours before admission.

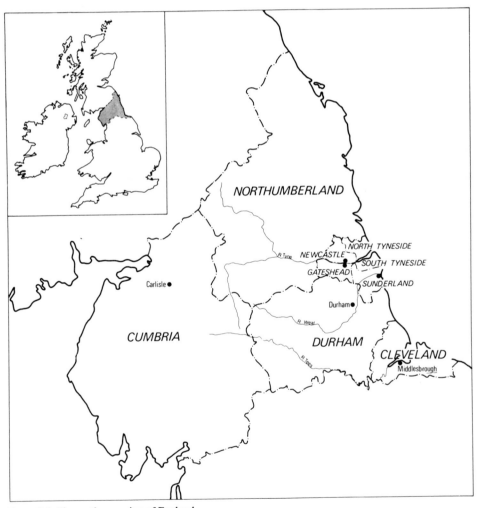

Figure 2.1. The northern region of England.

All patients included in the study were admitted to one ward and there was thus uniformity of management. There are few children in the series because policy dictates that they are admitted to the paediatric wards; the results of a companion study of 200 head injuries in children have already been published (Craft et al, 1972).

During the period of the study, 425 patients were admitted to the unit within 24 hours of receiving a head injury. Twenty-one of them died during the first 24 hours after admission. As our concern was with sequelae of head injury rather than with mortality and morbidity statistics, these patients were not included in the analysis; the initial cohort thus consisted of 404 patients. Apart from the early deaths, a further 32 patients died before discharge and thus the final cohort for follow-up study was reduced to 372 patients.

During the period in hospital, patients were seen at least once a day for the purposes of the study. Soon after admission, as much information as possible was obtained about the nature of the accident, its cause and circumstances. In the case of road accidents, inquiry was made about the type of vehicle involved, about the state of the road and the weather, about seat belts and about lighting conditions. Clinical information as to site and severity of head injury, presence or absence of skull fracture, level of consciousness and general neurological status was also recorded and notes were kept of all investigations performed together with their results.

Throughout the period in hospital serial neurological and psychological examinations were recorded by a single examiner (N.E.F.C.). Then, prior to discharge, further detailed assessments were made and noted. These included: neurological and psychological symptom check lists; a psychometric evaluation including the Roth Hopkins memory, concentration and information test; and standard neurological and psychological examinations. In addition, patients and their relatives were interviewed by a social worker who was specially appointed for the study. She sought detailed information concerning the socioeconomic status of the patient prior to injury, explored in as much detail as possible the previous health record and the educational and occupational history, and tried to establish a personality rating against which postaccident comparisons could be made.

A standard follow-up programme was conducted and attempts were made to reassess survivors at intervals of six months, one year and two years after discharge from hospital. Where patients were unable or unwilling to attend hospital for follow-up, home visits were undertaken and vigorous efforts were made to track down defaulters. Some patients moved away from the region and, where a home visit was not feasible, a detailed proforma was sent by post for completion and the help of a local physician or hospital was sought where necessary in an effort to keep the records up to date. At each follow-up visit the neurological and psychological assessments that had been made at the time of discharge were repeated and a further socioeconomic evaluation was carried out by the social worker. Attention was paid in particular to changes in the patients' economic status and also to any changes in mood, personality and general behaviour pattern that could be judged from personal observation and by enquiry from the family. Particular note was made of loss of working time since the accident, and all details of claims, benefits, pensions and compensations were recorded.

All information obtained during the period in hospital, on discharge and at follow-up visits was entered on special proformas designed for computer analysis. Ultimately, the data were transferred to punch cards. The computer analysis was carried out by Mr. Angus McNay and his colleagues in the statistical department of the Regional Health Authority in Newcastle using an IBM. 627X computer.

Some of the basic information relating to the 404 patients included in the study is presented in the tables. Table 2.1 shows the age and sex distribution of the total cohort.

The general composition of the group is very similar to that recorded in many of the retrospective studies referred to in Chapter One. It simply confirms the high percentage of young males admitted to hospital as a result of head injury.

The distribution according to social class of the head injury patients has been compared with that of the general population (Table 2.2). There is a slight preponderance of members of the upper two social classes in the head injury group; this runs contrary to the findings of Kerr et al (1971) and Baldwin (quoted by Field, 1976). In Australia, Selecki et al (1967) reported that an unexpectedly high proportion of patients with head injury were labourers and craftsmen, and Klonoff (1971) in Canada reported that children suffering from head injury tended to come from families of lower occupational status.

Table 2.1. Age and sex distribution of patients with head injury (Newcastle study).

Age (years)	Male	Female	Total
15—19	69	31	100
20—29	74	13	87
30—39	38	8	46
40—49	36	9	45
50—59	30	17	47
60—69	26	17	43
70—79	12	16	28
80 +	2	6	8
Total	*287*	*117*	*404*

As was to be expected, the follow-up information was not complete. In spite of vigorous efforts to trace all those involved, there were a few who could not be found. Of the 372 patients in the follow-up cohort, 258 faithfully attended all three scheduled visits. An additional 78 patients attended on two occasions, whilst for 15 patients information is available from only one follow-up examination. In 21 cases no follow-up information was available. Five of these patients had been visiting Newcastle when head injuries occurred; after discharge, they moved back to their own homes away from the region. None of them replied to repeated letters and we were unable to elicit any information from their general practitioners. Three of those lost to follow-up were local Newcastle patients who could not be traced despite repeated visits to their home addresses. The remainder of those who were untraced fell into the category of vagrants, most of whom were alcoholics.

Instead of counting the defaulters, we can put the follow-up figures in the more positive terms of attendance and say that, of the total of 372, 338 patients were seen at

Table 2.2. Social class distribution of patients with head injury (Newcastle study).

Registrar General's Classification	Head injury cases		General Population (%)
	(Nos.)	(%)	
I	26	21	12.3
II	60		
III	182	45	52.3
IV	70	17	21.6
V	66	17	13.8
Total	*404*	*100*	*100*

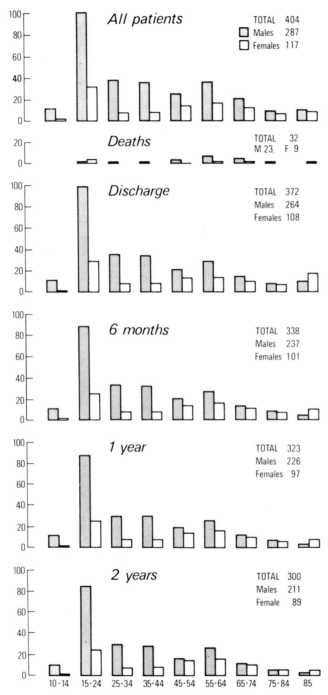

Figure 2.2. Age and sex distribution of patients in the study.

the six-month follow-up visit, 323 at the one-year visit and 300 at the two-year visit. The age and sex distributions of the follow-up groups remained fairly constant, indicating that there was no selective drop-out of a particular sex or age group (Figure 2.2).

In this chapter we have given an outline of the methods used in the prosecution of the study and a breakdown of the patient population on admission, at discharge and at follow-up. The clinical data recorded on these patients will be discussed in later chapters but first the causes of head injury, both in the present study and in other recorded series, will be considered.

REFERENCES

Craft, A. W., Shaw, D. A., Cartlidge, N. E. F. (1972) Head injuries in children. *British Medical Journal*, **iv**, 200-203.
Denny-Brown, D. (1945) Disability arising from closed head injury. *Journal of the American Medical Association*, **127**, 429-436.
Field, J. H. (1976) Epidemiology of head injuries in England and Wales. London: Her Majesty's Stationery Office.
Jennett, B., Teasdale, G., Braakman, R., Minderhoud, J. & Knill-Jones, R. P. (1976) Predicting outcome in individual patients after severe head injury. *Lancet*, **i**, 1031-1034.
Kerr, T. A., Kay, D. W. K. & Lassman, L. P. (1971) Characteristics of patients, type of accident, and mortality in a consecutive series of head injuries admitted to a neurological unit. *British Journal of Preventive and Social Medicine*, **25**, 179-185.
Klonoff, H. (1971) Head injuries in children — predisposing factors, accident conditions, accident proneness, and sequelae. *American Journal of Public Health*, **61**, (12), 2405-2417.
Russell, W. R. (1932) Cerebral involvement in head injury. *Brain*, **55**, 549-603.
Selecki, B. R., Hoy, R. J. & Ness, P. (1967) A retrospective study of neuro-traumatic admissions to a teaching hospital. 1. General aspects. *The Medical Journal of Australia*, **2**, 113-117.

CHAPTER THREE

Causes of Head Injury

Chance plays a major part in most accidents but in some at least there are recognizable predisposing factors. Such factors may be inherent in the individual as a reflection of his or her physical or psychological make-up. They may, on the other hand, be environmental and beyond the control of the individual. The intrinsic factors can vary from time to time; swings of mood, worries and preoccupations, even phases of the menstrual cycle may influence the susceptibility of an individual to an accident. McFarland, Moore and Warren (1955) have developed this concept of accident proneness which is with some of us all of the time whilst in others it is a variable phenomenon. The relationship between personality and proneness to road accidents is of particular interest and Whitlock (1971) has attempted to correlate a tendency to aggressive behaviour in motor-vehicle drivers with a predisposition to accidents.

The role of environmental factors in the causation of accidents is in many cases obvious. Occupation stands out as a prime factor, but such things as the games we play and the recreations we follow may also influence our chances of having an accident. Factors like these are bound to create a sex difference and indeed the patterns of accidents vary considerably between men and women. Since road accidents are so common, the time we spend in our motor cars must influence our chances of injury; our alcohol intake is another variable of considerable significance. Since so many of these variables can be related to differing social patterns, it is clear that correlations between categories of accident and socioeconomic groupings are bound to emerge.

Of all the factors that have a bearing on the types of accident that occur, the most important one is age. Man has been said to have 'seven ages' that mark his passage through life. We would not presume to suggest that these were defined with special reference to his proneness to head injury but, nevertheless, particular accident patterns do predominate during certain phases of life. The 'mewling and puking' infant, for instance, is certainly at risk of head injury. He faces two main hazards: being dropped or being battered (or, as we prefer to call it nowadays, non-accidentally injured). As he gets a little older, and moves into the second phase, the risk of battering continues but other new hazards emerge. He begins to crawl and then to walk and, as he becomes more adventurous, his chances of injury increase. Jackson and Wilkinson (1976) have drawn attention to our extraordinary disregard of the most fundamental aspects of safety for children in this one-to-five-years age group. Even in buildings and play areas which are specially designed for children there are often features that are very unsafe and fail to take into account the remarkable propensity of small children for climbing (Figure 3.1). Conventional playgrounds have their own inherent risks, and swings are responsible for a good many mishaps.

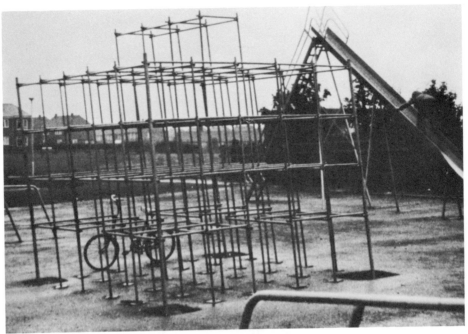

Figure 3.1. Hazards of the playground.

In the next phase, from five to ten years, the range of activity increases. At this age, children climb trees and slide down bannisters. They start to ride bicycles and ponies and are out on the roads as pedestrians, often unaccompanied. There is a marked increase in the risk of head injuries in this age group; the peak incidence of road accidents in children is in their seventh and eighth years.

Over the next five years, from age ten to 15, the pattern remains much the same except that assaults become rather more common. The danger to the 'whining schoolboy' is not so much from parents as from schoolmates. Sporting injuries also begin to increase and unsupervised games result in a good many accidents (Figure 3.2).

The next age covers adolescence and early adulthood. The male at least may be 'sudden and quick in quarrel' and there is a further increase in the incidence of assaults (Figure 3.3). There is a greater risk of serious sporting injuries; it is also in the period from 15 to 25 years that road accidents, fewer of them now pedestrian, reach their highest proportions. The latter are certainly responsible for the great majority of

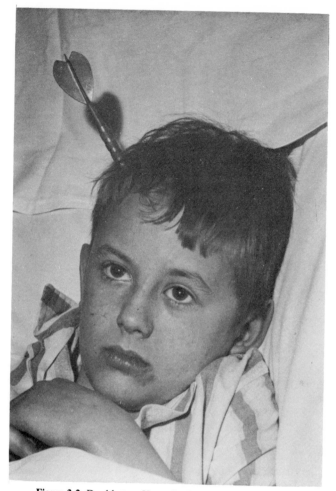

Figure 3.2. Double top. Hazards of unsupervised games.

hospital admissions with head injury in this particular age group. Table 3.1 is a summary of five hospital studies in which causes of injury in adults have been analysed. Road accidents account for approximately half of the cases of head injury in all series. There are differences in the ways in which the data were collected in the various studies, and this accounts for some of the apparent discrepancies, but by and large all the studies within the series are broadly comparable.

The sixth of our seven ages runs throughout adult life to the age of retirement. During this long period, road accidents continue at a fairly steady level which is somewhat lower than that in young adults. Industrial injuries occur at a fairly even rate, and accidental falls become more common as people get older. For the purposes of head injury classification our last age runs from retirement through to the 'second childishness and mere oblivion' of the more famous literary prototype. Even the very elderly continue to go out and about and as pedestrians they run the serious risk of being knocked down, but accidental falls at home represent the greatest danger.

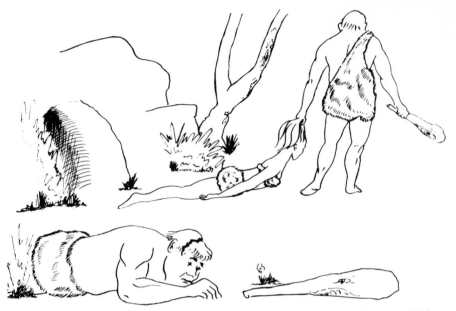

Figure 3.3. Head injury from assault. With kind permission of Dr. Ned I. Chalat of Detroit, Michigan and the editor of *The Laryngoscope*.

The foregoing section is a rough sketch of the pattern of head injuries as they occur from infancy to old age. Let us look now in more detail at some of the characteristics of the 404 head injuries that comprise the Newcastle series. As indicated in Chapter One, our study was not concerned with children and all patients had to have reached the age of 15 years to be eligible for inclusion. However, a separate but broadly comparable study of children has been carried out in Newcastle (Craft, Shaw and Cartlidge, 1972). This survey included 200 children who were admitted to hospital with head injury. Thirty-three per cent were injured as a result of a road accident and 27.5 per cent had had an accident at home, usually a fall. Accidents at school accounted for 12.5 per cent of the total, and seven per cent of all the injuries were the result of an assault. Amongst the children involved in road accidents were some no more than three years old; the peak incidence for this kind of injury was between six and seven years. At this age the majority were pedestrians. In older children bicycle injuries began to take an increasingly significant toll (Craft, Shaw and Cartlidge, 1973). Injuries occurring at school were spread throughout the whole school age range and in most instances they resulted from sporting accidents or from unsupervised play. Assaults occur mainly at the extremes of childhood; the youngest ones are injured by their parents whilst the older children are hurt through fighting one another.

Table 3.2 lists the main categories of injury in our series and shows the distribution in each according to age. The nature of each category is self-evident, except in the case of the miscellaneous group which included five patients. Two of these suffered their head injuries by walking into obstacles that they did not notice. One was an unfortunate youth who had been watching his local football team; as he left the ground, a flagpole was blown over by a gust of wind, it hit him on the head and rendered him unconscious. The remaining two had head injuries resulting from attempted suicide. One was a student who shot himself through the mouth with a .22 revolver. The bullet passed up between his frontal lobes and he did not even lose consciousness. He afterwards suffered from

Table 3.1. Causes of injury in adults.

Author and country	Population	Age range and number	Road accident (%)	Domestic or falls (%)	Industrial (%)	Assault (%)	Sport (%)	Other (%)
Rowbotham et al (1954) England	Newcastle General Hospital admissions	13 yrs and over n = 1000	44	8 (domestic)	31	3	3	11
Klonoff and Thompson (1969) Canada	Visits to emergency department —admissions to neuro-surgical ward (22% transferred cases)	16 yrs and over n = 351	44	20 (falls)	10	13	5	8
		16 yrs and over n = 279	53	23 (falls)	11	4	3	6
Kerr, Kay and Lassman (1971) England	Newcastle General Hospital admissions (20% transferred)	15 yrs and over n = 474	48	16 (domestic)	14	13	3	6
Barr and Ralston (1964) Scotland	Peripheral general hospital admissions	all ages n = 532	67	11 (domestic)	9	2	11 (including children at play)	—
Steadman and Graham (1970) England	Cardiff Royal Infirmary admissions (7% transferred)	all ages n = 484	45	14 (domestic)	9	7	3	19

Table 3.2. Accident categories and distribution according to age (Newcastle study).

	15—19	20—29	30—39	40—49	50—59	60—69	70—79	80+	Total
Road accidents	53	46	20	14	19	19	18	2	191
Work accidents	7	9	11	12	12	6	0	0	57
Sports accidents	10	2	1	0	0	0	0	0	13
Assaults	12	16	8	3	4	2	1	0	46
Accidental falls	15	13	6	16	11	16	9	6	92
Miscellaneous	3	1	0	0	1	0	0	0	5
Total	*100*	*87*	*46*	*45*	*47*	*43*	*28*	*8*	*404*

persisting cerebrospinal fluid rhinorrhoea and required a subfrontal exploration to close the dural tear; but in the long run he made a good recovery and his only neurological defect was bilateral anosmia. The other case of attempted suicide was a psychotic female who threw herself from a cliff and suffered multiple fractures in addition to her head injury.

Table 3.3. Categories of accidents and sex distribution (Newcastle study).

	Male	Female	Total
Road accidents	126	65	191
Work accidents	50	7	57
Sports accidents	10	3	13
Assaults	41	5	46
Accidental falls	56	36	92
Miscellaneous	4	1	5
Total	*287*	*117*	*404*

The figures in Table 3.2 are not adjusted to take into account the population at risk; nevertheless the extremely high incidence of road accidents, sporting injuries and assaults is immediately apparent. Head injuries from accidents are, of course, of major importance throughout all age groups, and work accidents are very evenly distributed up to retiring age. Accidental falls are also well represented throughout and their incidence is particularly conspicuous in the very old.

Table 3.4. Categories of accidents and socioeconomic groupings (Newcastle study).

	I		II		III		IV		V		Total
	(nos.)	(%)	(nos.)	(%)	(nos.)	(%)	(nos.)	(%)	(nos.)	(%)	(nos.)
Road accidents	16	8	41	21	78	41	29	16	27	14	191
Work accidents	0	0	2	3	28	49	18	32	9	16	57
Sports accidents	3	23	3	23	6	46	0	0	1	8	13
Assaults	0	0	2	4	18	39	8	18	18	39	46
Accidental falls	7	8	11	12	49	53	14	15	11	12	92
Miscellaneous	0	0	1	20	3	60	1	20	0	0	5
Total	*26*	*7*	*60*	*15*	*182*	*45*	*70*	*17*	*66*	*16*	*404*

Table 3.5. Seasonal and sex distribution of accidents (Newcastle study).

Month	Male	Female	Total (nos.)	Total (%)
January	21	9	30	7
February	26	21	47	10
March	34	9	43	9
April	31	14	45	10
May	24	13	37	8
June	32	8	40	9
July	37	10	47	10
August	28	8	36	8
September	20	5	25	5
October	10	5	15	7
November	8	4	12	5
December	15	11	26	12

When we look at a breakdown of the accident categories in relation to sex (Table 3.3) we find a male predominance throughout. Indeed, there are nearly two and a half times as many injuries in males as in females and the most striking sex differences are in the categories of assaults and accidents at work. A crude analysis of accidents in relation to socioeconomic group is shown in Table 3.4, but again the figures are unadjusted. The Table does however indicate a higher incidence of road accidents in the upper three socioeconomic groups, and sport injuries are virtually restricted to these groups. There does not appear to be any relationship between accidental falls and socioeconomic groups; assaults, however, are much more common in the lower categories.

The timing of injuries is often of interest and the influence of environmental or social factors may be detected. Klonoff and Thompson (1969) found that patients with head injury were most commonly brought to hospital between 5 p.m. and midnight and they commented on a rising incidence at weekends. They also reported a slightly higher frequency of head injuries during the spring months. Partington (1960) found that childhood injuries were twice as common in summer as in winter. Our own figures for injuries in adults show no striking seasonal influence (Table 3.5), but the weekend effect is apparent, peak admission figures being on Fridays and Saturdays (Table 3.6). This high incidence of weekend injuries affects males and females alike (Table 3.7). Finally, there is in Table 3.8 a breakdown of accidents according to the sex of the

Table 3.6. Day and age distribution of accidents (Newcastle study).

Day	Below 20	20—29	30—39	40—49	50—59	60—69	70—79	80+	Total
Monday	11	15	9	10	5	6	5	1	62
Tuesday	13	8	2	8	7	4	5	0	47
Wednesday	14	4	6	6	5	6	2	0	43
Thursday	13	9	6	4	10	5	5	2	54
Friday	19	16	11	2	6	11	2	2	69
Saturday	14	17	9	8	7	10	8	2	75
Sunday	16	18	3	7	7	1	1	1	54
Total	100	87	46	45	47	43	28	8	404

Table 3.7.   Day and sex distribution of accidents (Newcastle study).

Day	Male	Female	Total
Monday	46	16	62
Tuesday	34	13	47
Wednesday	30	13	43
Thursday	38	16	54
Friday	48	21	69
Saturday	50	25	75
Sunday	41	13	54
Total	*287*	*117*	*404*

individual and the time of day of the accident's occurrence. There is a strikingly high incidence in both males and females between 10 p.m. and midnight; the inescapable conclusion is that this peak has something to do with drinking habits. It is not altogether clear why there should be so many more accidents in males in the early afternoon than in the forenoon but it is possible that here too alcohol is a relevant factor, and fatigue may also play a part.

In the remaining paragraphs of this chapter we will consider some factors relevant to the particular categories of accident, but we will omit road accidents, which are considered in the next chapter.

Table 3.8.   Hour and sex distribution of accidents (Newcastle study).

Hour	Male	Female	Total
00.01—01.00	6	1	7
01.01—02.00	8	0	8
02.01—03.00	4	2	6
03.01—04.00	4	0	4
04.01—05.00	2	0	2
05.01—06.00	2	1	3
06.01—07.00	0	1	1
07.01—08.00	8	1	9
08.01—09.00	6	5	11
09.01—10.00	6	5	11
10.01—11.00	16	9	25
11.01—12.00	8	9	17
12.01—13.00	9	6	15
13.01—14.00	13	3	16
14.01—15.00	16	4	20
15.01—16.00	17	5	22
16.01—17.00	26	7	33
17.01—18.00	10	8	18
18.01—19.00	12	6	18
19.01—20.00	9	6	15
20.01—21.00	8	5	13
21.01—22.00	11	2	13
22.01—23.00	25	15	40
23.01—24.00	50	10	60
Not recorded	11	6	17
Total	*287*	*117*	*404*

ACCIDENTAL FALLS

If we exclude road accidents, the commonest cause of head injury at all ages is an accidental fall. At the extremes of life this cause predominates (Craft, Shaw and Cartlidge, 1972; Cummins and Potter, 1970). There is in our series a surprisingly high incidence of accidental falls in women (Table 3.3) and about half of the falling accidents occur in the home. These accidental falls at home turn out to be more common in the lower three socioeconomic groups, and middle-aged women are particularly prone to injury from this cause. Of the total of 92 patients whose head injury resulted from a fall, 14 had had a faint or a fit and one had had a stroke.

Alcohol plays an important part in the causation of head injuries resulting from accidental falls. Thirty-four of the 92 patients who fell had recently taken alcohol. Forty-three of them fell inside the home and, of these, 12 had had alcohol. Altogether, ten of the falls (eight men and two women) were due to profound intoxication, but milder degrees undoubtedly contributed to many of the others. There are, of course, many hazards such as unlit stairs, uneven pavements and icy patches on the roads which may topple the sober as well as the inebriated. The confusion and unsteadiness of the very elderly are certainly common causes of mishap.

WORK ACCIDENTS

The preceding section refers to accidental falls in the home, in the streets and in public places. The figures do not include head injuries resulting from falls at work. These are in fact quite common and, of the 57 injuries in our series that occurred at work, no fewer than 23 were due to falls. In the majority of cases these were falls from a height and of course this represents a hazard in a great many industries and service occupations. The great majority of injured workers were males, 50 out of a total of 57, and only six of them had consumed alcohol before the accident. Only in about half of the injuries was it possible to understand precisely the cause of the accident and to apportion blame. In 15 instances the accident was due to negligence on the part of the injured party, and in 16 there was negligence on the part of someone else.

SPORTS ACCIDENTS

A significant number of accidents occur in the course of sporting activities of one sort or another. In most instances it is the young from the upper social classes that are affected. The principal offending sports are rugby football, soccer and horse riding (Figure 3.4); in our series they were the cause of 13 cases (3.2 per cent). The medical literature contains a number of interesting reviews of head injuries resulting from sports. Haddon (1966) has considered sports in general and Unterharnscheidt (1970 and 1975) has written about boxing and other sports. Foster, Leiguarda and Tilley (1976) have discussed the problem of brain damage in steeplechase jockeys.

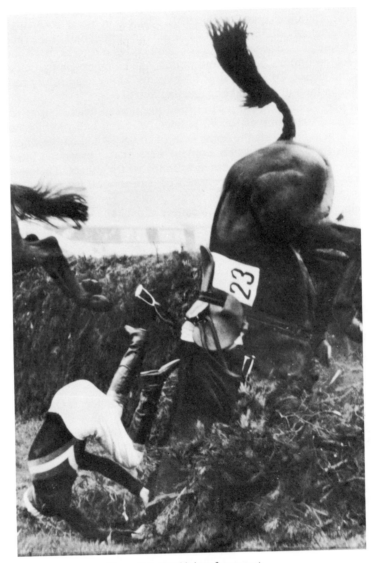

Figure 3.4. Head injury from sport.

ASSAULTS

In our series the assault figures were somewhat alarming. There were in all 46, representing 11.4 per cent of the total. Thirty-five of these patients had taken alcohol and about half of the assault injuries were a direct result of a bar-room brawl. The injuries varied from the impulsive attack of a psychotic patient with an axe to the more 'conventional' blow on the head with a beer bottle. There were five women amongst those who were assaulted and in each case it was the husband who was the assailant. In our series the assault cases were almost entirely confined to the lower three socio-economic groups. We had two patients who were admitted twice to the study; in both cases the history was one of repeated fights resulting in head injury.

REFERENCES

Barr, J. B. & Ralston, G. J. (1964) Head injuries in a peripheral hospital, *Lancet,* **ii,** 519-522.

Craft, A. W., Shaw, D. A. & Cartlidge, N. E. F. (1972) Head injuries in children, *British Medical Journal,* **iv,** 200-203.

Craft, A. W., Shaw, D. A. & Cartlidge, N. E. F. (1973) Bicycle injuries in children. *British Medical Journal,* **iv,** 146-147.

Cummins, B. H. & Potter, J. M. (1970) Head injuries due to falls from heights. *Injury,* **2,** 61-64.

Foster, J. B., Leiguarda, R. & Tilley, P. J. B. (1976) Brain damage in National Hunt jockeys. *Lancet,* **i,** 981-983.

Haddon, W. (1966) Principles in research on the effects of sports on health. *Journal of the American Medical Association,* **197,** 163-166.

Jackson, R. H. & Wilkinson, A. W. (1976) Why don't we prevent childhood accidents? *British Medical Journal,* **i,** 1258-1262.

Kerr, T. A., Kay, D. W. K. & Lassman, L. P. (1971) Characteristics of patients, type of accident, and mortality in a consecutive series of head injuries admitted to a neurological unit. *British Journal of Preventive and Social Medicine,* **25,** 179-185.

Klonoff, H. & Thompson, J. B. (1969) Epidemiology of head injuries in adults — a pilot study. *Canadian Medical Association Journal,* **100,** 235-241.

McFarland, R. A., Moore, R. C. & Warren, B. A. (1955) Human variables in motor vehicle accidents. Harvard School of Public Health, Boston.

Partington, M. W. (1960) The importance of accident proneness in the aetiology of head injuries in childhood. *Archives of Diseases of Children,* **35,** 215-223.

Rowbotham, J. F., McIver, I. N., Dickson, J. & Bousfield, M. E. (1954) Analysis of 1400 cases of acute injury to the head. *British Medical Journal,* **i,** 726-729.

Steadman, J. H. & Graham, J. G. (1970) Rehabilitation of the head injured. *Proceedings of the Royal Society of Medicine,* **63,** 23-36.

Unterharnscheidt, F. J. (1970) About boxing: review of historical and medical aspects. *Texas Reports of Biology and of Medicine,* **28,** 421-492.

Unterharnscheidt, F. J. (1975) Injuries due to boxing and other sports. In *Handbook of Clinical Neurology* (Ed.) Vinken, P. J. & Bruyn, G. W. Volume 23, Chapter 26, Oxford: North-Holland Publishing.

Whitlock, F. A. (1971) *A Study in Social Violence.* London: Tavistock Publications. New York: Barnes and Noble.

CHAPTER FOUR

Road Accidents

The possible dangers of traffic on the highways were recognized from the earliest days in motoring history. Indeed, legislation introduced in the 19th century to protect the public from this new menace was so restrictive that it considerably retarded the development of the self-propelled vehicle. As early as 1831 the English Parliament enacted laws that virtually eliminated the 'horseless carriage' which at that time was driven by steam. One of the most discouraging pieces of legislation for the enthusiastic engineers of the day was the 'Red Flag Law' which required that a man precede the vehicle carrying a red flag by day and a red lantern by night. Furthermore the tolls on roads and bridges for self-propelled vehicles were raised to prohibitive levels. It was not until 1896 that the laws in England became rather less restrictive and the development of the internal combustion engine seemed a more worthwhile investment. It should be noted, however, that in that same year two deaths resulting from motor vehicle accidents were registered in Great Britain and three years later the first death from the same cause was registered in the United States. Ever since then the mortality figures have gone on rising and by 1951 the United States had recorded their millionth road traffic death.

Increasing alarm over the hazards of the roads has been reflected in the expanding volume of legislation that has been seen over the years. A great many sensible measures have been introduced but their effects have been overwhelmed by the relentless growth of the motor car and its ever-increasing role as an instrument of destruction. Amongst the many legislative innovations a few stand out as landmarks. The Road Traffic Act of 1930 introduced driving tests for some licence holders and made third-party insurance compulsory. The Act of 1934 imposed a 30 m.p.h. speed limit in built-up areas, and introduced pedestrian crossings. At the same time new regulations came in about windscreen wipers and about the use of safety glass. Between 1949 and 1954 there were further regulations about pedestrian crossings, and brakes on bicycles became compulsory. The Highways Act was introduced in England in 1959 and this brought in some new rules about motorways and the use of double white lines in the centre of roads. Between 1961 and 1963 compulsory vehicle testing was introduced and in 1967 the fitting of seat-belts to new cars became a legal requirement. About this time there was growing public awareness of the dangers of drinking and driving and in England it became an offence to attempt to drive a vehicle with a blood alcohol level of over 80 mg/100 ml. In 1969 it became compulsory to have vehicles tested annually if they were three years old or more; recently new regulations have come into force about vehicle design and it has become illegal for motorcyclists to ride without safety helmets.

These are but a few of the many regulations that have been introduced in the United Kingdom. It is perhaps significant that although the population and the number of vehicles on the road has tended to rise in recent years, there has been a levelling off in the number of road accidents and resultant casualties. These facts are illustrated in Figure 4.1 which is taken from the 1978 Road Accident Report for Great Britain (Department of Transport, 1980). Nevertheless, during the ten years prior to publication of the report, nearly 100 000 people were killed or seriously injured on the roads per annum. It has been estimated that road accidents in Great Britain cost more than one million pounds each day (Department of Transport, 1976) and in the United States a cost of 10 billion dollars per annum has been quoted (Haddon, 1971). In Canada the annual cost of road accidents has been estimated at one billion dollars per annum (Thompson and Klonoff, 1975). Comparative figures for road deaths in different countries for the year 1973 are shown in Table 4.1.

Of the 404 head injuries in the Newcastle series, 191 resulted from road accidents. As was mentioned in the last chapter (see Table 3.2), the highest incidence was in drivers in their teens and twenties. Also, twice as many males as females were involved: Table 4.2 shows details of the precise role of the injured person involved in the accident: the male to female ratio varies somewhat in the different categories. Males constitute the great majority of lone car drivers who are injured and also the majority of injured motorcyclists and pedal cyclists. Equal numbers of men and women are injured as pedestrians and, as might be expected, a disproportionate number of women are injured as passengers in cars.

As has already been stated, the great majority of road accidents occur in the younger age groups. Accidents involving pedestrians are the only exceptions to this general rule (Table 4.3). All age groups are equally likely to be involved in road traffic accidents, but it is as pedestrians that the great majority of people over the age of 70 are injured.

Overall there is a higher incidence of road accidents in the higher socioeconomic groups (see Table 3.4). If we consider again the precise role of the injured person in relation to social class distribution in the Newcastle series (Table 4.4) we see that pedestrian accidents are more common in the lower socioeconomic groups; the same is true in the case of motorcycle accidents. Presumably car ownership equates to some extent with social class so it is not surprising therefore that the majority of injured drivers and passengers belong to the upper three socioeconomic groups.

In the following section we will consider in more detail some of the factors involved in the causation of road accidents.

THE INDIVIDUAL AND ROAD ACCIDENTS

Whitlock (1971) has suggested that traffic accidents are largely an expression of violence on the roads and are simply one facet of aggression in our society. In support of his argument he demonstrates that correlations exist between road deaths and other

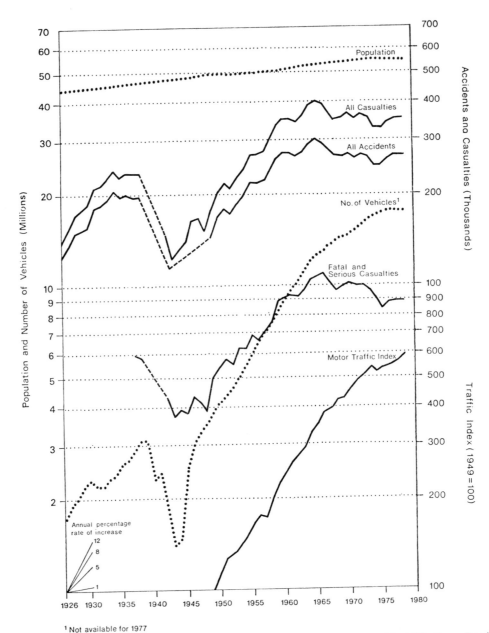

Figure 4.1. Population, vehicles licensed, accidents, traffic and casualties, 1926—1978. From Road Accidents Great Britain 1978 (1980), with kind permission of the Controller of Her Majesty's Stationery Office. (Logarithmic scale.)

Table 4.1. Road deaths and death rates in various countries: 1973.

Country	Number of road deaths	Vehicles per 100 population	Road deaths per 100 000 population	Road deaths per 10 000 vehicles	Car user deaths per 100 million car miles	Pedestrian deaths per 100 000 population
Great Britain	7 406	31	14	4	3	5
Australia	3 675	46	28	7	:	6
Austria	2 469	30	37	12	11	10
Belgium	2 905	32	30	9	(10)	(8)
Canada	6 706	46	30	7	(3)	6
Czechoslovakia	2 073	18	19	10	:	6
Denmark	1 132	30	23	8	(3)	5
Federal Republic of Germany	16 302	30	26	9	5	7
Finland	1 086	28	23	8	3	6
France	15 469	46	32	7	9	6
German Democratic Republic	2 122	31	14	5	:	4
Hungary	1 831	14	18	13	10	6
Irish Republic	592	19	20	10	3	7
Italy	10 728	35	21	6	(4)	5
Netherlands	3 092	40	23	6	4	4
New Zealand	843	54	29	5	:	5
Norway	511	31	13	4	3	4
Poland	4 200	9	16	17	18	7
Portugal	1 312	11	21	19	(12)	8
Spain	4 764	17	18	10	14	5
Sweden	1 177	33	14	4	3	3
Switzerland	1 451	39	23	6	4	7
United States of America	55 800	57	25	4	3	5
Yugoslavia	4 377	8	21	27	23	7

Numbers within brackets indicate the figures for 1972.

Table 4.2.   Sex distribution of road accidents (Newcastle study).

	Male	Female	Total
Lone driver	20	1	21
Accompanied driver	12	3	15
Front passenger	9	14	23
Rear passenger	11	9	20
Pedestrian	35	32	67
Motorcyclist	30	3	33
Bicyclist	8	0	8
Motorcycle pillion rider	1	3	4
Total	*126*	*65*	*191*

accidental deaths, suicides, deaths from violence, rape, robbery and indeed all violent crime encountered by the police. Clearly no one would expect any single factor to be responsible for the road death epidemic but it does seem likely that personality factors do play a significant role in accidents. Accident proneness has already been suggested as a possible factor of relevance and it does seem that certain groups of individuals, particularly those with poor personal and social adjustment, have an unexpectedly high incidence of road accidents. It should be said that a case against the notion of accident proneness as a personality trait and as a cause of road accidents has been put by Norman (1962), and the matter is still open to debate. It is of note that in our own series no one was involved in a road accident more than once.

It is generally accepted that illness and infirmity bear a relationship to accident rates. Our own figures show only the effect of age upon pedestrian deaths but, it has been estimated, on the basis of much more extensive studies, that between one and two in a thousand road accidents can be attributed to acute or chronic illness in car drivers (Grattan and Jeffcoate, 1968; Bull, 1970; Ysander, 1970). A difficult question arises as to what disabilities, in terms of category and severity, should constitute a barrier to the possession of a driving licence. If we accept that even a small number of accidents are caused by drivers having myocardial infarcts, it could be argued that patients with known coronary artery disease should be banned from driving. At the same time this would obviously be a very discriminatory regulation and it would impose great hardship. The same argument could apply to a great many other conditions, and the potential complexities of the medical regulations are unimaginable. Because epilepsy is relatively easy to define and because it represents such an obvious potential source of accident, the

Table 4.3.   Age distribution of road accidents (Newcastle study).

	15—19	20—29	30—39	40—49	50—59	60—69	70—79	80 +	Total
Lone driver	1	12	4	1	2	1	0	0	21
Accompanied driver	3	7	4	0	0	1	0	0	15
Front passenger	8	8	3	0	2	0	1	1	23
Rear passenger	7	3	2	2	1	2	3	0	20
Pedestrian	11	7	6	5	10	14	12	1	67
Motorcyclist	16	7	1	5	3	1	0	0	33
Bicyclist	4	1	0	0	1	0	2	0	8
Motorcycle pillion rider	3	0	0	1	0	0	0	0	4
Total	*53*	*46*	*20*	*14*	*19*	*19*	*18*	*2*	*191*

Table 4.4. Social class distribution of road accidents (Newcastle study).

	I	II	III	IV	V	Total
Lone driver	5	7	8	1	0	21
Accompanied driver	2	4	9	0	0	15
Front passenger	3	7	8	2	3	23
Rear passenger	1	8	8	3	0	20
Pedestrian	2	11	24	12	18	67
Motorcyclist	3	2	15	9	4	33
Bicyclist	0	2	4	0	2	8
Motorcycle pillion rider	0	0	2	2	0	4
Total	*16*	*41*	*78*	*29*	*27*	*191*

law is clear about the situation of the epileptic in relation to driving; likewise visual impairment, which is easily identified and measured, is catered for in the rules. It has been suggested that the granting of driving licences should involve regular and relatively frequent medical examinations. However, when the logistics of this proposition are examined, it is clear that routine examination of all potential motor drivers would sterilize a substantial part of our medical resources. In spite of this difficulty, it is clear that further problems have to be tackled in relation to medical and psychiatric illnesses and the control of driving licences. On the other side of the coin, it must be stated that a number of studies suggest that mild mental and nervous illness, poor sight and hearing, and moderate physical disability have little effect on the frequency of accidents, possibly due to the fact that those affected take greater care to avoid mishaps (Bull, 1970; Eelkema et al, 1970).

A study of patients discharged from a state mental hospital in the United States showed a higher incidence of road accidents than in a group of controls (Eelkema et al, 1970). A study in California (quoted by Norman, 1962) showed that drivers suffering from chronic illnesses such as diabetes, hypertension or renal disease, had twice the accident rate of those without these diseases. In a survey of a thousand deaths and consecutive admissions to hospital after traffic injury, Jamieson and Tate (1966) found evidence of six acute medical events which were thought to have predisposed to the road accidents. There were three probable seizures, one cerebral haemorrhage, one subarachnoid haemorrhage and one myocardial infarction. Five of the individuals involved were car drivers and one was a motorcyclist. Only three of these events were thought likely to have been predictable on the basis of routine medical examination; the authors concluded that less than 0.3 per cent of the licence holders involved in the accidents would have been barred from driving had they had routine medical examinations. It therefore seems unlikely that medical selection of drivers will make a significant impact on the accident rates. Certainly ill-health could not be held responsible for any of the accidents that occurred in our own series.

It is commonly held to be true that if a driver becomes fatigued he is progressively more liable to accident, although the proportion of road accidents which are directly due to fatigue in the driver is unknown. Fatigue is recorded by the police as a relevant factor in less than one per cent of all road accidents in the United Kingdom causing personal injury (Norman, 1962), although this may well be an underestimate. Two patients in the present study were injured after the driver of a car fell asleep at the wheel. Both of these patients were rear-seat passengers in a car in which the driver was killed instantly at the time of the accident, whereas a front-seat passenger received virtually no injury.

ALCOHOL AND DRUGS

Alcohol is perhaps the most important single factor which affects human behaviour and which has been identified as important in serious accidents, in homicide and in suicide. It has been shown many times that the drinking driver is particularly prone to accident, and data in support of this come from a great many countries. Pearson (1957) in Australia found that, out of 200 fatal-road-accident victims, 39 per cent had an alcohol concentration in the blood of at least 100 mg/100 ml and 24 per cent had 200 mg/100 ml or more. Even more striking are the figures quoted by Jamieson and Tate (1966). Of 41 drivers killed in road accidents and regarded by the police as being responsible for the accident, 41 per cent had a blood alcohol concentration of 100 mg/100 ml or more, whereas no alcohol was found in the blood of a group who were involved in accidents but who were not held responsible by the police. This sort of difference was not found amongst pedestrians involved in accidents and the same study showed that only 16 per cent of passengers who were killed in accidents had alcohol levels of 100 mg/100 ml or greater.

In the United States of America the story is very much the same. Haddon and Bradess (1959) found that, out of 83 drivers killed in single vehicle accidents, 49 per cent had blood alcohol levels of 150 mg/100 ml or more at death. Comparable figures could be quoted from studies carried out in many other parts of the world including Great Britain. Legislation introduced here in 1967 enabling the prosecution of drivers with blood alcohol levels in excess of 80 mg/100 ml resulted in a striking reduction in the number of serious and fatal accidents involving cars.

Table 4.5 presents data concerning alcohol intake in relation to type of road accident and the role of the injured person in the accident. We do not have comprehensive data on individual blood levels but we know that over 30 per cent of those injured had recently consumed alcohol and it is interesting to note that the highest figures are amongst lone drivers. If we group together all drivers with head injury we find that 60 per cent of them had been drinking. A relatively small proportion of people injured whilst riding a motorcycle had been taking alcohol. As might be expected, the relationship between alcohol consumption and road accidents is most apparent at the weekends; national figures show a very striking increase in the number of accidents associated with drinking on Fridays, Saturdays and Sundays. Our own figures show the same trend.

The role of drugs in the causation of road accidents is less clear (Ashworth, 1975), although evidence suggests that they may play an increasing part in the future as larger

Table 4.5. Alcohol intake and type of road accident (Newcastle study).

	Yes	No	Total
Lone driver	13	8	21
Accompanied driver	7	8	15
Front passenger	7	16	23
Rear passenger	7	13	20
Pedestrian	27	40	67
Motorcyclist	6	27	33
Bicyclist	2	6	8
Motorcycle pillion rider	1	3	4
Total	*70*	*121*	*191*

numbers of people are taking tranquillizers and sedatives. Hossack (1972) reported on a study in Australia involving 400 people killed in road accidents. Seven per cent of the drivers who died had amphetamine, barbiturate or bromide in their blood. Apart from this study there are few data on this subject and certainly in our own series we have no evidence that drug intoxication played a part in any of the accidents.

ENVIRONMENT

There is a strong association between road accident rates and the weather and state of the roads. Yearly statistics are produced in the United Kingdom (Department of Transport, 1976 and 1980) and these detail many aspects of road surface, weather, and lighting conditions in relation to road accidents. It has been shown for instance that accident rates fall by about 30 per cent when lighting is installed on previously unlit roads. One particular example of the importance of street lighting in the reduction of accidents can be quoted. In order to conserve fuel during the emergency period in the winter of 1973/4, local authorities in the United Kingdom were urged in November and December 1973 to reduce the consumption of electricity for street lighting. The restrictions lasted until 12th March 1974 when full lighting was restored to all roads. During the period of saving there was a deterioration in the casualty record in darkness as compared with daylight, particularly at nonjunction sites and this deterioration was substantially greater than would have been expected from past trends. The recognition of the adverse effects of road surface has influenced changes such as the introduction of motorways, crash barriers, hazard-warning lights and speed limits on poor road surfaces.

In our own series of 191 road accidents, 97 occurred during daylight hours and 94 at night. Thirty-three of the 94 night-time accidents were on roads with street lighting; 50 of the accidents occurred whilst it was raining, one during fog, one whilst it was snowing and the remainder under fine conditions. The road surfaces were described as dry in 136 of the accidents, wet in 46 and icy or snow-covered in 9.

THE MACHINE

It is only in recent years that legislation has been passed in the United Kingdom to ensure that vehicles on the road are mechanically sound and contain protective devices to safeguard drivers and passengers. Primary safety is achieved as a result of good engineering design and efficient vehicle maintenance (Thomas, 1970). Secondary safety is defined as the attempt to reduce or prevent injuries when crashes do occur.

Recognition of the importance of primary safety in the United Kingdom has led to compulsory annual tests for all cars that are more than three years old (Transport Act and Traffic Act, 1962). Perhaps the first application of secondary safety measures was that of Sir Hugh Cairns in relation to motorcycle accidents. Cairns found that despatch riders in the army had a high mortality rate after accidents, and this led him to recommend the compulsory wearing of crash helmets; a striking decrease in mortality followed. Secondary safety features in the car now include a variety of accident restraint systems: collapsible steering wheels, safety doors, protected fuel systems, etc.

Of these perhaps the most effective is the safety belt. The main function of safety belts is to protect their wearers from head injury as a result of striking the windscreen (Grime, 1968) and a number of studies have shown that wearing them significantly decreases the mortality and morbidity rates in road accidents (Galasko and Edwards, 1975). In the United Kingdom this has led to legislation to ensure that all new cars now produced have seat belts fitted.

Our own figures provide striking confirmation of the effectiveness of seat belts. Out of 58 car drivers or front seat passengers admitted during the period of our study with a head injury, not one was wearing a seat belt. As our study covered all possible admissions with head injuries over a 21 month period it provided strong presumptive evidence that wearing a seat belt at the time of an accident gives good protection. Of the people in our study injured in a motorcycle or scooter accident, 50 per cent were wearing a crash helmet, indicating that this of course does not give total protection from head injury. Our data, however, would support the view that crash helmets reduce the severity of head injuries, as the only person who died following a motorcycle accident was not wearing a helmet.

There has been an interesting suggestion that automobiles may, in general, contribute indirectly to road accidents because of their effects on the atmosphere. Ury, Perkins and Goldsmith (1972) reported that in Los Angeles there was an association between the level of air pollution, as measured by carbon monoxide levels, and the frequency of motor vehicle accidents. It may be, of course, that the correlation depends on the fact that carbon monoxide levels are likely to be higher when there is a lot of moisture in the atmosphere with accompanying changes in visibility.

It is clear that road accidents are an all-too-common cause of head injury and we have to remember that the Newcastle data that we present here take no account of the early fatalities that resulted from accidents. The figures the world over are really quite appalling and it is an interesting commentary on our society that, whilst we are shocked by an isolated disaster claiming a handful of lives, we come to terms quite readily with a daily death toll on the roads of such enormous proportions. A great deal of information is accumulating on a wide range of factors that play a part in the causation of accidents. It would seem that this is an area in which preventive medicine could play a highly significant role, given the social and political will to take positive steps to tackle the problems of road accidents which claim so many young lives.

REFERENCES

Ashworth, B. M. (1975) Drugs and driving. *British Journal of Hospital Medicine,* February, 201-204.
Bull, J. P. (1970) Epidemiology of road accidents. *British Journal of Hospital Medicine,* October, 437-440.
Department of Transport (1976) *Road Accidents, Great Britain, 1974.* Her Majesty's Stationery Office, London.
Department of Transport (1980) *Road Accidents, Great Britain, 1978.* Her Majesty's Stationery Office, London.
Eelkema, R. C., Brosseau, J., Kishnick, R. & Magee, C. (1970) A statistical study on the relationship between mental illness and traffic accidents — a pilot study. *American Journal of Public Health,* **60,** 459-469.
Galasko, C. S. B. & Edwards, D. H. (1975) The use of seat belts by motor car occupants involved in road traffic accidents. *Injury,* **6,** 320-324.
Grattan, E. & Jeffcoate, G. O. (1968) Medical factors and road accidents. *British Medical Journal,* i, 75-79.
Grime, G. (1968) Information on injuries obtained from reports of accidents to car occupants wearing seat belts. *Conference on Road Safety — Brussels.*
Haddon, W. (1971) A logical framework for categorising highway safety phenomena and activity. *Journal of Trauma,* **11,** 65-69.
Haddon, W. & Bradness, A. (1959) Alcohol in the single vehicle fatal accident — experience in West Chester County, New York. *Journal of the American Medical Association,* **169,** 1587-1593.

Hossack, D. W. (1972) Investigation of 400 people killed in road accidents with special reference to blood alcohol levels. *Medical Journal of Australia,* **2,** 255-258.

Jamieson, K. G. & Tate, I. A. (1966) Traffic injury in Brisbane. *The National Health and Medical Research Council Report Series No. 13,* Canberra, Australia, 1966.

Norman, L. G. (1962) Road traffic accidents. *Public Health Papers No. 12. World Health Organisation, Geneva.*

Pearson, A. T. (1957) Alcohol and fatal traffic accidents. *The Medical Journal of Australia,* **2,** 166-167.

Thomas, L. H. (1970) Safer cars. *British Journal of Hospital Medicine,* October, 451-454.

Thompson, G. B. & Klonoff, H. (1975) Epidemiology of head injuries, Chapter 2. In *Injuries of the Brain and Skull,* Part I, Volume 23, *Handbook of Clinical Neurology* (ed.) Vinken, P. J. & Bruyn, G. W. Amsterdam, Oxford: North Holland Publishing Company. New York: American Elsevier Publishing.

Ury, H. K., Perkins, N. M. & Goldsmith, J. R. (1972) Motor vehicle accidents and vehicular population in Los Angeles. *Archives of Environmental Health,* **25,** 314-322.

Whitlock, F. A. (1971) *A Study in Social Violence.* London: Tavistock Publications. New York: Barnes and Noble.

Ysander, D. (1970) Sick and handicapped drivers: A study on the risks of sudden illness at the wheel, and on the frequency of road accident and traffic offences in chronically sick, disabled and elderly drivers. *Acta Chirurgica Scandinavica* (Supplement **409**).

CHAPTER FIVE

The Medical and Social Consequences of Head Injury

Attention has been drawn in previous chapters to some of the crude statistics of head injury. In this chapter we propose to look more specifically at its consequences: to analyse the patterns of mortality and morbidity and to consider also the social and economic deprivations that so often result. In later chapters we shall go a step further and consider particular sequelae, such as motor paralysis and epilepsy, and attempt to establish their incidence and the factors which determine their prognosis.

DEATHS FROM HEAD INJURY

The most clearly defined and immutable outcome of head injury is death. As might be expected, an analysis of the mortality figures mirrors fairly accurately the general epidemiological profile of head injury. The greater number of deaths in males than in females corresponds to the higher incidence of head injury in the male, and the number of deaths that result from road accidents is a fair reflection of the contribution that such accidents make to the total incidence of head injury. The rule does not hold good when we consider the factor of age in relation to head injury mortality. Although half of those admitted to hospital with head injury are under the age of 20 years, a much higher proportion of deaths occur in people over the age of 40.

A great many head injury deaths are sudden. About 30 per cent of those who are going to die do so before reaching hospital and probably a further 20 per cent die in casualty departments before full resuscitative measures can be implemented. Another 40 per cent or so die sooner or later after reaching the wards. This leaves only about ten per cent of fatal cases who will die after discharge from the initial hospital. Of these, one per cent will finally succumb in long-stay psychiatric hospitals and another one per cent will die after a prolonged period in what Jennett and Plum have called the 'persistent vegetative state'. This term, which is a useful one and which we will use again, describes patients who 'never regain recognisable mental function, but recover from sleep-like coma in that they have periods of wakefulness when their eyes are open and move; their responsiveness is limited to primitive postural and reflex movements of the limbs, and they never speak' (Jennett and Plum, 1972).

These figures are, of course, approximations. They must vary from place to place depending on admission and discharge policies, factors which of themselves influence the overall mortality figures in different centres. Such figures quoted from a number of reported series are shown in Table 5.1.

Table 5.1. Mortality from head injury in hospital-based studies.

Authors	Period of study	Number of cases	Age range	Case fatality rates (%)
Rowbotham et al (1954)	1945—51	1000	13 years and over	17.5
		400	0-12 years	8.5
Lewin (1954)	1948—53	1000 (direct admissions)	not stated	7.1
		280 (transferred in)	not stated	12.2
Steadman and Graham (1970)	1958	484 (7% transferred in)	all ages	1.9
Barr and Ralston (1964)	1957—61	532 (2% transferred out)	all ages	4.7
Kerr et al (1971)	1963—64	474 (20% transferred in)	15 years and over	10.8

According to the rules of entry into our Newcastle study, it was necessary for a patient to have survived for 24 hours after admission to hospital to be included in the survey. Of the 404 patients who fulfilled this criterion, 32 died whilst still in hospital — a mortality rate of 7.9 per cent, as is shown in Table 5.2. In this table the mortality for each cause of head injury is analysed. Nearly half of those admitted to the study had had road accidents, and the mortality in this group was substantially higher than in the other categories of head injury. Although they were not eligible for the study, records were kept of patients who died within 24 hours after admission to the neurosurgical unit. During the period of the study there were 16 patients and the overall mortality including these was calculated at 11.4 per cent.

Table 5.2. Mortality and cause of head injury (Newcastle series).

	Alive	Dead		Total
Road accident	170	21	(11%)	191
Work	53	4	(7%)	57
Sport	13	0		13
Accidental fall	85	7	(7.6%)	92
Assault	46	0		46
Miscellaneous	5	0		5
Total	*372*	*32*	*(7.9%)*	*404*

MORBIDITY IN SURVIVORS

Whilst head injury mortality figures for the population are relatively easy to calculate, accurate statistical information on the numbers of brain-damaged survivors is much more difficult to come by. Such figures as are available are generally based on extrapolations from the individual experience of a single centre to the population at large. London (1967) calculated that head injury inflicted serious handicap on 1 000 people in Britain each year, with half of them permanently incapable of a return to work of any sort. Lewin (1970) has estimated that in the same population approximately 1 500 individuals will suffer permanent major disability because of head injury. Nine hundred of these will be capable of employment although at a diminished level; the remaining 600 will be virtually unemployable. A detailed head injury study in Glasgow (Jennett et al, 1976) has shown that between one and two per cent of patients still unconscious more than six hours after head injury will be left in the 'persistent vegetative state'. A further five to eight per cent will remain severely disabled and incapable of living alone.

In recent years there has been increasing social and political awareness of the needs and hardships of the handicapped in our communities. A few years ago an attempt was made in Britain to estimate the size of the problem by the launching of the National Social Survey of the Handicapped and Impaired. The figures derived from this survey, quoted by Field (1976), indicated that in 1968-69 there were 12 000 head-injured people over the age of 16 living in private households and suffering from disabilities severe enough to limit their ability to work or to get about independently. It was thought that a great many of these had relatively minor deficits which need not necessarily have been so disabling, the implication being that with better social and medical provision their lives might be improved. Nevertheless, the survey confirmed that there is a large pool of morbidity within the community that is all too easily forgotten and that represents economic loss for the community as well as hardship for the individual.

LIFE EXPECTANCY AFTER HEAD INJURY

It is generally accepted that, whilst early mortality from head injury is so high, there is surprisingly little reduction in life expectancy for those who survive. This obviously has medicolegal importance, there being so many claims for compensation for individuals who have suffered head injury. The severity of the injury and its immediate sequelae obviously have some bearing on the life expectancy. For instance, those who recover only as far as the 'vegetative state' have a very poor outlook and the majority will die within months, or occasionally years, of their injury. This correlation between life expectancy and severity of injury seems to hold good even in the less severe grades. Amongst patients who recover sufficiently to return to their homes, it is the most seriously injured who have the diminished life expectancy. Hillbom (1960) produced figures to show that late mortality increases significantly with severity of head injury. Fahy, Irving and Millac (1967) found in their study that 19 per cent of the early survivors of severe head injury had died by the time the follow-up was conducted after a six-year interval. Other studies have suggested a better long-term prognosis. Thus Miller and Stern (1965) studied a group of 100 patients at an interval of many years after their head injuries. The mean follow-up period was 11 years, and in this time only one patient had died as a result of the head injury. He had post-traumatic anosmia and accidentally gassed himself. Steadman and Graham (1970) studied 484 patients five years after head injury and found that none had died from their injury after discharge from hospital.

In order to construct proper life tables for head injury it would be necessary to have accurate information on patients going back a great many years. Unfortunately, such data are not available for civilian survivors of head injury, but the careful recording of brain wounds in war has enabled Walker (1971) to construct life tables. Walker did not give details of the criteria of entry to his study, but the brain injuries that his patients had suffered were generally more severe than those usually seen in civil hospital practice. His tables showed a reduction in life expectancy, at all ages, of men who had survived head injury, and the reduction was particularly marked in those whose head injury had resulted in epilepsy. The difference between life expectancy of those with and without head injury became increasingly obvious over the age of 50; at the age of 75 life expectancy was reduced by 3.3 years in those whose head injury had not resulted in epilepsy and by 4.9 years in those with epilepsy.

There are a variety of ways in which further clues about head injury morbidity may be obtained. Hospital in-patient statistics provide information as to bed usage. In 1972 the average number of hospital beds occupied daily by patients with head injury in England and Wales was 1809. This represented one per cent of all hospital bed usage, excluding maternity. In our Newcastle study we found that it was possible to discharge the majority of patients after a relatively short period in hospital. The duration of stay is analysed in Table 5.3 and it will be seen that only ten per cent of patients had to remain in hospital for more than two weeks. All of the 32 patients who died in hospital did so within the first week after admission. Whilst length of stay in any one hospital following head injury is obviously influenced to a great extent by that hospital's admission policy, the overall pattern is fairly constant, and our own Newcastle figures are very similar to those for the rest of England and Wales (Field, 1976).

In the United Kingdom, statistics are available on certified absence from work due to sickness or injury and they provide a further commentary on head injury morbidity. They have the great advantage that they tell us something of what happens after patients leave hospital. They do have their limitations and unfortunately they apply only to the working population; furthermore they take no account of periods of sickness of less than four days. Field (1976) reports the figures for England, Scotland and Wales for the year 1969/70. The median duration of time off work was 18 days

Table 5.3. Length of hospitalization (Newcastle series).

Length of time	Male	Female	Total
24 hours	32	3	35
1—2 days	60	35	95
2—3 days	48	20	68
3—4 days	23	8	31
4—5 days	16	9	25
5—6 days	17	5	22
6—7 days	11	9	20
7—8 days	12	4	16
8—14 days	40	12	52
15—21 days	8	7	15
Three weeks	20	5	25
Total	*287*	*117*	*404*

for patients with fracture of the skull or face bones and 13 days for patients with intra-cranial injury without fracture. During the year in question, 1 748 000 days were lost as a result of head injury and this amounts to 2.1 per cent of days lost as a result of industrial injuries of all types.

In the Newcastle study, records of attendance at work were kept during the follow-up period and the results are summarized in Table 5.4. Patients are categorized according to the percentage of time lost from work since the last review and the percentage of patients in each category has been analysed at follow-up intervals of six months, one year and two years. Between the time of discharge from hospital and the first six-month follow-up visit only ten per cent of patients had had no time off work and almost 20 per cent of them had been off work throughout the entire period. By the one-year follow-up, 61 per cent of those seen had had no time off work since the six-month visit, and by the two-year follow-up 66 per cent of those seen had had no time off work during the preceding year. At the one-year and two-year follow-up visits, 16 per cent and 14 per cent respectively had been off work continuously.

Table 5.4. Time away from work (Newcastle series).

Time away from work as a percentage of the time since last seen	Period of follow-up		
	6 months (%)	1 year (%)	2 years (%)
None	10	61	66
10%	29	10	14
10—50%	29	9	4
50—90%	13	4	2
100%	19	16	14

SOCIAL AND ECONOMIC SEQUELAE

The figures in the preceding sections tell us something of the impact of head injury in social and economic terms, but few studies have been designed specifically to examine the problem. The study of Dresser et al (1973) did attempt to examine particu-larly the achievement in terms of employment of a group of men who had suffered head injury. The subjects were 864 American servicemen who had been injured during the Korean war, and the study was carried out some 15 years after the time of injury. When they were assessed, subjects were aged between 30 and 40 years. The authors constructed a control group consisting of 120 individuals from the same Service units who had escaped without head injury. At the time of follow-up only 75 per cent of the study subjects were working, in contrast to 95 per cent of the controls. Comparison also showed that in the head-injured group there had been less regularity in the patterns of employment and promotions had been less frequent.

An assessment of the economic status of all patients entering the Newcastle study was made by our social worker at about the time of their admission to hospital. She recorded absolute figures on income but also noted particularly whether the economic status of the individual was rising, falling or about stationary at the time of the accident. It was found that 70 per cent were in the static group whilst 28 per cent had rising expectations and two per cent were declining in economic status. At the six-month follow-up the percentage of those in the declining group had risen to 13; 22 per cent were thought to be improving their economic status whilst 65 per cent were static. By the end of a year the figures were: 68 per cent static, 26 per cent rising and six per cent falling. By the time the two-year follow-up point was reached, the percentages in the three categories were virtually back to where they were at the time of admission to hospital. At the follow-up visits the patients were asked for details of their occupations; it was found that at six months after injury 15 per cent of those working were in lighter jobs than before injury. This figure declined very gradually; at one year it had fallen to 14 per cent and by the end of two years 10 per cent were still in lighter jobs than they had been in before their injury.

COMPENSATION

Occasionally we read in the press of large sums of money being awarded to individuals in compensation for a head injury that they have suffered, but relatively little information is available as to the general level of compensation that is paid. Before considering in detail such information as is available concerning the sums of monetary compensation for the head injured, it is perhaps appropriate for us to outline the spectrum of benefits, allowances and compensations that may be claimed in the United Kingdom.

Private compensation claims may be made under British Common Law through the offices of solicitors or lawyers. Under these circumstances awards of compensation are generally made only if negligence is proved, and solicitors' and other legal fees must be paid whether the claimant wins or loses his case. All employed working individuals who become incapable of work because of illness may claim 'sickness benefit'. Those absent from work because of an industrial injury may claim 'industrial injury benefit'; a 'loss of earnings claim' may be made under both these benefits. Each is payable for a maximum of six months. Inability to return to work beyond this period entitles an individual who was receiving sickness benefit to claim 'invalidity' benefit, and 'disablement benefit' may be paid in the same circumstances to someone who has previously been in receipt of 'injury benefit'. Disablement benefit may be paid as a regular pension or a lump sum gratuity, depending on the degree of disability. It is assessed by a medical board appointed for the purpose. Those injured as a consequence of criminal action may apply for compensation to the Criminal Injuries Compensation Board, a body which disburses lump sums from Government sources.

Information based on the payment of invalidity and disablement benefits is thus of limited value, as it applies only to those off work for more than six months. Field (1976) reported that, on a particular day in June 1973, there were 2 200 men who were receiving invalidity benefit in Britain because of head injury, and 1 200 of these had been off work for more than a year. The majority were men over the age of 55.

More-detailed information on compensation payments is available in the United States; Irving (1969) has quoted some interesting figures. Total compensation paid to all workers in 1966 under the compensation laws was approximately two billion dollars; 665 million dollars of this was for individual and hospital costs and 1 300 million was for wage compensation. Of these vast sums, 1 257 million dollars was said to come from private firms whilst 454 million came from state funds and 264 million from private insurance schemes. These figures relate to accidents of all sorts, and head injury accounted for seven per cent of them. That seven per cent absorbed eight per cent of the compensation total.

In the Newcastle study, information was sought as far as was possible on compensation claims and receipts. Table 5.5 gives an indication at the three follow-up intervals of the numbers of patients receiving monies by way of compensation from our normal public sources. Figures on private compensation claims are summarized in Table 5.6. The number of claims is high. At six-month follow-up 88 (26 per cent) of the head-injured patients had processed a private compensation claim, and by the end of the two-year follow-up as many as 33 per cent had claims pending.

Table 5.5. Compensation and other monetary claims from public sources.

	6 months	1 year	2 years
Disability pension	10	13	13
'Loss of earnings' claim	7	9	15
Criminal Injuries Compensation			
Board claim	5	7	9
Total of patients	338	323	300

In the course of this chapter we have attempted to describe the effects of head injury in terms of mortality, morbidity and social and economic deprivation. Although some of the figures are surprisingly high it is probable, nevertheless, that we under-estimate the magnitude of the problem; the true amount of suffering both by patients and relatives as the result of head injury is probably immeasurable. In the following chapters we shall turn to the more specific medical sequelae and, on the basis of our Newcastle figures, try to detail as precisely as possible the incidence of the various disabilities that result from head injury and to comment on the factors that produce them and that determine their capacity for recovery and response to treatment.

Table 5.6. Private compensation claims (Newcastle series).

	Number of claims		Total number of patients
	No.	(%)	
6 months	88	(26)	338
1 year	100	(31)	323
2 years	100	(33)	300

REFERENCES

Barr, J. B. & Ralston, G. J. (1964) Head injuries in a peripheral hospital. *Lancet*, **ii**, 519-522.
Dresser, A. C., Meirowsky, A. M., Weiss, G. H., McNeel, M. L., Simon, G. A. & Caveness, W. F. (1973) Gainful employment following head injury; prognostic factors. *Archives of Neurology*, **29**, 111-116.
Fahy, T. J., Irving, M. H. & Millac, P. (1967) Severe head injuries. *Lancet*, **ii**, 472-479.
Field, J. H. (1976) *Epidemiology of Head Injuries in England and Wales.* H.M. Stationery Office.
Hillbom, E. (1960) After effects of brain injuries. *Acta Psychiatrica Neurologica Scandinavica* (Supplement 34).
Irving, J. G. (1969) Impact of insurance coverage on convalescence and rehabilitation of head injured patients. *The Late Effects of Head Injury.* (Ed.) Walker, A. E., Caveness, W. F. & Critchley, M. Chapter 48. Springfield, Illinois, U.S.A.: C. C. Thomas.
Jennett, B. & Plum, F. (1972) Persistent vegetative state after brain damage. *Lancet*, **i**, 734-737.
Jennett, B., Teasdale, G., Braakman, R., Minderhoud, J. & Knill-Jones, R. (1976) Predicting outcome in individual patients after severe head injury. *Lancet*, **i**, 1031-1034.

Kerr, T. A., Kay, D. W. K. & Lassman, L. P. (1971) Characteristics of patients, type of accident, and mortality in a consecutive series of head injuries admitted to a neurological unit. *British Journal of Preventive and Social Medicine,* **25,** 179-185.

Lewin, W. (1954) Head injuries in civil practice. *Proceedings of the Royal Society of Medicine,* **47,** 865-869.

Lewin, W. (1970) Rehabilitation needs of the brain injured patient. *Proceedings of the Royal Society of Medicine,* **63,** 8-12.

London, P. S. (1967) Some observations on the course of events after severe injury of the head. *Annals of the Royal College of Surgeons of England,* **41,** 460-479.

Miller, H. & Stern, G. (1965) The long-term prognosis of severe head injury. *Lancet,* **i,** 225-229.

Rowbotham, G. F., McIver, J. N., Dickson, J. & Bousfield, M. E. (1954) Analysis of fourteen hundred cases of acute injury to the head. *British Medical Journal,* **i,** 726-729.

Steadman, J. H. & Graham, J. G. (1970) Rehabilitation of the brain injured. *Proceedings of the Royal Society of Medicine,* **63,** 23-36.

Walker, A. E., Leuchs, H. K., Lechtape-Grüter, H., Caveness, W. F. & Kretschman, C. (1971) Life expectancy of head injured men with and without epilepsy. *Archives of Neurology,* **24,** 95-100.

CHAPTER SIX

The Neurological Features of Head Injury Coma

The most common, immediate and obvious consequence of a head injury is an alteration in the level of consciousness. This may vary from 'being dazed for a moment or two' to a state of irrecoverable coma. Severity of injury is often gauged by the patient's level of consciousness, and judgements on immediate chances of survival and long-term prospects of recovery are greatly influenced by readings of this barometer of brain activity. Familiarity with the physical signs that characterize the unconscious state and discernment of their fluctuations are thus essential to the understanding and management of head injuries.

The brain may be damaged in a number of ways: three types of head injury — closed, penetrating and crush — are distinguished according to the mechanics of the trauma. Closed head injuries, which are the most common, result from falls or blows where the head is in sudden contact with another object and there is mechanical displacement of the brain within the skull as a result of acceleration or deceleration forces. Penetrating head injuries result from missiles such as bullets or sharp instruments. Crush injuries, as the name implies, occur when the head is subjected to two or more forces acting in opposite directions. These three types of injury produce their adverse effects in different ways. For detailed accounts of the mechanics of brain damage due to head injury, the reader is referred to the excellent contributions to the Conference on Head Injury held in Chicago in 1966 (Caveness and Walker, 1966).

In the Newcastle study there were five examples of crush injury and 22 of penetrating injuries. The remainder were closed injuries, which are certainly the most common type in civilian practice; emphasis will be on these in the consideration of neurological sequelae.

THE ACUTE EFFECTS OF HEAD INJURY

There are wide variations in the early manifestations of head injury both in the degree of disturbance of consciousness and in the extent of alteration of other neural activities. The traditional approach to the classification of altered states of consciousness after head injury is outlined in the Medical Research Council War Memorandum No. 4 (1941). The type and severity of the injury are the principal determinants of the early manifestations and, following the example of Symonds (1937), it may be helpful to indicate the sort of clinical effects that may accompany injuries of varying degrees of seriousness.

At one end of the scale is the minor injury that might result from a 'knock-out blow' in boxing. The victim slumps to the ground and lies inert. Within seconds, or at most a minute or two, he gets up and staggers around. At this stage he is usually able to answer simple questions and recovery may be quick enough for him to box on within the count. Alternatively, he may take a few minutes to return to apparent normality only to realize later that he has no memory for events immediately following the blow, indicating a period of post-traumatic amnesia.

In a slightly more severe injury the patient will fall to the ground and lie motionless. There may be temporary arrest of respiration and the legs may give a few myoclonic jerks. Examination at this stage will probably show areflexia, dilatation of the pupils and an absent lash reflex. Provided that respiration resumes almost immediately, the patient will soon begin to move his limbs and he may become restless and even violent. This stage may be limited in duration to a few minutes and he should soon begin to obey commands and answer simple questions, although he may still be confused and unaware of his surroundings. This last state may last for a few hours, but by the next day the patient will be normal except for a period of post-traumatic amnesia of up to about 12 hours.

The third example is of a more severe head injury with loss of consciousness for 24 hours or more. In this case recovery will naturally take longer and there may be a prolonged period of post-traumatic delirium. During this phase the patient may be totally irrational and difficult to manage, with a tendency to fight with his medical attendants. Eventually he will pass into a more rational though confused state persisting for up to two days; in cases of such severity there is usually post-traumatic amnesia for up to a week. Patients showing this degree of disturbance have often had a traumatic subarachnoid haemorrhage. As a general rule the longer the period of unconsciousness the more prolonged are the stages of recovery, including the period of post-traumatic amnesia. There are, of course, exceptions to the rule and the only certainty is that, after injuries of this severity, there is a more or less regular sequence of recovery of cerebral function from the lowest level to the highest.

Finally, there are the really severe cases in which patients may show the features of so-called 'primary brain-stem injury', which will be discussed further in Chapter Seven. Injuries of this severity most commonly result from road accidents where the head may be dashed against the windscreen or strike the road after a person's ejection from the car. Such severe injuries may result in immediate decerebrate rigidity persisting, in fatal cases, up to the time of death. In such cases there will be abnormalities of respiration and of eye movements and pupillary reflexes. Not all patients with primary brain-stem injury die; some survive showing features of the persistent vegetative state (Jennett and Plum, 1972), while others may make better recoveries but not without residual neurological deficits.

Against the background of these brief paradigms of injury, we may look in detail at the neurological features of head injury coma.

NEUROLOGICAL SIGNS IN HEAD INJURY COMA

Careful documentation of clinical signs in comatose patients is of paramount importance (see Chapter 13). Most head injury units keep a chart by the bedside for ease of serial recording and to facilitate early recognition of change in level of consciousness, which may have practical importance in the detection of intracranial haematoma or oedema.

Various methods have been devised for the assessment of the unconscious patient. For our study in Newcastle we adopted the Ommaya Conscious Scale (Ommaya, 1966), which identifies five levels of consciousness (Table 6.1). The numbers of patients in the

Table 6.1. Ommaya Conscious Scale.

Level 1	Patient is orientated in time and place and is recording on-going events; that is, the state of normal consciousness defined operationally.
Level 2	Patient is talking and/or obeying commands but is disorientated and not recording on-going events.
Level 3	Patient is responding to stimuli with correct localization (purposeful), but is not obeying commands.
Level 4	Patient responds to stimuli without localization, that is, non-purposeful reflex or decerebrate response only.
Level 5	Totally unresponsive to all stimuli.

different categories on admission are shown in Table 6.2, with a breakdown according to death or survival. Forty-three patients were still in coma at the time of their admission to the study and more than half of them died. The Ommaya Scale is relatively crude but it does provide some guide to severity and, from the data in Table 6.2, it is clear that the outcome is worst in patients entering the study at the lowest levels of consciousness.

Since the Newcastle study was undertaken, a new method of assessing levels of consciousness has been proposed by Teasdale and Jennett (1974). It is based on a major head injury study initiated in Glasgow and carried out in collaboration with other centres in Europe and the United States. It has the merit of simplicity and has been widely adopted both in the routine management of head injury and also in a computerized system of outcome prediction; the latter is based on a data bank

Table 6.2. Conscious level (Ommaya scale) on admission in the Newcastle series.

Ommaya scale	Outcome		
	Survived	Died	Total
1	272	2	274
2	81	6	87
3	18	15	33
4	1	9	10
5	0	0	0
Total	*372*	*32*	*404*

comprising serial observations on 1000 cases of severe head injury (Jennett et al, 1979). The method can be operated satisfactorily by trained nursing staff (Teasdale, Galbraith and Clarke, 1975) and its reliability has been confirmed in an observer variation study (Teasdale, Knill-Jones and Van der Sand, 1978).

hierarchical scoring of responses to appropriate stimuli in three separate areas of function — eye-opening, limb movement and verbal response (Table 6.3).

Table 6.3. Glasgow Coma Scale.

Eye-opening	Spontaneous
	To speech
	To pain
	None
Motor response	Obedience to commands
	Localization of pain
	Withdrawal
	Flexion to pain
	Extension to pain
	None
Verbal response	Orientated
	Confused conversation
	Inappropriate words
	Incomprehensible sounds
	None

In each category, responses to appropriate stimuli are graded from the highest to the lowest.

EYE-OPENING

Failure to open the eyes or to do so only in response to a painful stimulus is a feature of coma. Spontaneous or noise-induced eye-opening occurs in normal arousal and it differentiates sleep from coma. In general, achievement of spontaneous eye-opening after coma implies recovery, but there may be an exception in prolonged comatose states in which a patient may remain unresponsive yet show a return of spontaneous eye-opening. This state of wakefulness without awareness characterizes the so-called 'vegetative state' (Jennett and Plum, 1972). Usually it takes two or three weeks for a comatose patient to enter the state and it is certainly rare within a week of injury. Fortunately it is uncommon, for the condition can be tragic and prolonged. It is not always permanent; one of the cases in the Newcastle study illustrates progression from the vegetative state to a higher level of recovery.

The patient (Case 229) was a 39-year-old man who was knocked down by a motor car. On admission to hospital he was breathing spontaneously but was completely flaccid. Bilateral temporal burr holes were made and small, scarcely significant haematomas were evacuated from the subdural space. On the day after admission he was still deeply unconscious and had Cheyne—Stokes respiration. The respiratory rate was increased to 45 per minute by painful stimuli, and these also provoked decerebrate responses. Deep tendon reflexes were pathologically brisk and the plantar responses were extensor. Pupillary and corneal reflexes were preserved and iced water in the ears produced appropriate deviation of the eyes to either side, although responses were modified by a right sixth-nerve palsy. For three days thereafter the patient's condition remained virtually unchanged and he continued to have spontaneous attacks of decerebrate rigidity ('tonic fits'). Over the next few days these diminished in intensity and the right sixth-nerve palsy cleared. The corneal reflexes became excessively brisk and there was a suggestion of grimacing in response to pain. Ten days after admission occasional opening of the eyes was noticed and by two weeks the pattern of spontaneous eye-opening was clearly indicative of regular sleep-wake cycles. The patient was now in the vegetative state, and flexor rather than extensor tone predominated in the arms. Within three weeks he was swallowing and moving his tongue spontaneously at times when the eyes were open, but there was no response at all to verbal commands. It was not until four weeks after the injury that a movement of the left hand in response to command was observed.

Six months after injury the patient had slight voluntary movement of the left arm and leg but there was no movement on the right side. He could not walk. He could just communicate but his speech was grossly impaired; he had marked emotional lability and was not capable of coherent conversation. He was discharged to long-term care and there was no subsequent recovery.

Limb Movements

Assessment of reflex motor responses, muscle tone, deep tendon reflexes and plantar responses are important elements in the examination of the patient in coma after head injury. Decerebrate or extensor responses and extensor tone may persist from the time of injury to death, and these are features in patients with so-called 'primary brain-stem injury'. In such patients tonic spasms may occur and these may be precipitated even by so light a stimulus as the draught from an open door. In addition to extensor posturing of the arms and legs during a spasm, there may be extension of the head, an increase in respiration, excessive sweating and a change in blood pressure. The posturing is usually symmetrical and, though recovery is possible, the prognosis is poor if tonic spasms persist for more than 24 hours. It is perhaps worth noting that a decerebrate or extensor motor response is 'better' than no motor response at all.

Asymmetry of reflex motor responses is common in the unconscious patient. Reflexes in the arms may be brisker than in the legs or vice versa, and plantar responses may be flexor or extensor with no obvious significance attaching to their behaviour. The jaw jerk is sometimes excessively brisk in comparison with other tendon reflexes, but in our experience this has little significance. Four of our patients showed this phenomenon and two had jaw clonus, but none was left with a corticobulbar deficit.

The Glasgow head injury study has provided useful information on the relationship between early motor responses in coma and the final outcome of a case (Jennett et al, 1976); our experience has been consistent with theirs. We have found that total flaccidity indicates a poor prognosis. Ten patients who showed no motor response and had no muscle tone within the first 24 hours all died. Table 6.4 relates motor response in the first 24 hours to outcome and shows that the lower levels of response were associated with a poor prognosis in the Newcastle series.

Primitive facial reflexes, such as a pout, are not a feature of head injury coma. One of our patients in coma was observed to have a pout reflex, but was subsequently shown to be suffering from presenile dementia. When there is severe and permanent brain damage as a result of head injury a pout reflex may develop at a later stage, usually after three or four weeks, but it may subsequently disappear if improvement takes place.

Table 6.4. Motor responses during first twenty-four hours in relation to outcome (Newcastle series).

Response	Died	Survived	Total
Obeying commands, spontaneous movements	2	359	361
Localizing or flexor response	6	10	16
Decorticate response	1	1	2
Decerebrate response	13	2	15
Flaccid	10	0	10
Total	*32*	*372*	*404*

A discrepancy between motor responses and other expressions of conscious level should alert the examiner to the possibility of an associated spinal cord injury. All together there were ten spinal fractures in our series, but only two patients had evidence of cord damage. There were an additional seven patients thought to have signs of spinal cord lesions in association with their head injuries. In each case x-rays showed pre-existing cervical spondylosis, suggesting that this had been responsible for contusion of the cervical cord.

Verbal Response

Absence of verbal or vocal responsiveness is part and parcel of the definition of coma. One of the pitfalls is, of course, the possibility that disturbance of verbal response may be an expression of dysphasia rather than coma. In such a case, the examiner is usually alerted by the discrepancy between the level of verbal response and that of other responses when a painful stimulus is applied.

One of the patients (Case 303) in our series, a man of 28, fell while drunk and suffered injury to the right frontal region and the right side of his face. At the time of admission he was restless and made occasional spontaneous semipurposive movements of both arms and legs. There was no response to verbal stimuli; to pain, he opened his eyes and showed bilateral localizing motor responses but there was no verbal response. By the third day his movements included spontaneous eye-opening, a localizing motor response to pain and occasional motor responses to vigorous vocal commands. Despite this, the only verbal response was an incomprehensible moan. By the sixth hospital day the patient had begun to speak and it became apparent that he was dysphasic.

Brain-stem Reflexes

Although spontaneous and reflex eye movements are not an integral part of the Glasgow Coma Scale, careful observation of them can provide additional information on both the site and the severity of brain damage in the unconscious patient. Roving movements of the eyes, either conjugate or disconjugate, are commonly seen when the closed eyelids are lifted. It is also common to see slight divergence of the eyes at rest. This is of no particular significance, being simply a manifestation of the normal degree of esophoria. Absence of spontaneous roving eye movements tends to be a bad sign. Amongst the 43 patients in our study who were comatose on admission, there were 19 with an absence of roving eye movements; seven of these died within 24 hours (Table 6.5).

Table 6.5. Brain-stem responses during first twenty-four hours in 43 comatose patients — in relation to outcome (Newcastle series).

	Died	Survived	Total
Absence of roving eye movement	7	12	19
Absence of oculocephalic reflexes	8	1	9
Absence of oculovestibular reflexes	6	0	6
Absence of corneal reflexes	7	2	9
Absence of pupillary reflexes	6	4	10

The reflex eye movements are of even greater value (Plum and Posner, 1976). The oculocephalic response, or doll's head manoeuvre, is induced by passive head rotation. It is the simplest test of reflex eye movement but is difficult to perform, particularly in intubated patients, and it requires keen observation. Normally, with horizontal head rotation to one side, the eyes deviate briskly and conjugately to the opposite side. Full conjugate excursion of the eyes indicates normal functioning of the labyrinths, eighth nerves, conjugate lateral gaze centres, medial longitudinal fasciculi, ocular motor nerves and ocular muscles. Absence of oculocephalic reflexes (i.e., eyes simply following the movements of the head) indicates a lesion of the brain stem in an unconscious patient. Responses are characteristically brisk in metabolic coma and depressed in coma due to drugs. Asymmetry of the oculocephalic responses may also indicate a brain-stem lesion. It is possible to test vertical reflex eye movements by neck flexion and extension, but responses are difficult to see.

The oculovestibular reflex, although it takes a little more time and trouble to perform, is easier to interpret than the oculocephalic and it is generally more reliable. It is induced by instillation of ice-cold water into the external auditory meatus, with the head at 30° to the horizontal. To be sure that the test has been adequately performed, up to 200 ml should be injected and observation should be continued for a full minute. In the normal conscious patient, nystagmus is produced, with the quick component away from the side of the stimulus. In the unconscious patient with an intact brain stem, there is tonic conjugate deviation to the side of the stimulus. In the presence of mild stem damage the tonic deviation may be disconjugate, and in the unconscious patient with severe brain stem damage, the responses are absent. This absence is a bad prognostic sign in patients in coma but it should be remembered that many drugs, particularly sedatives, may suppress the response; it should therefore be interpreted with caution in patients who have received medication. The reflex may also be absent in patients with middle ear disease or lesions of the eighth cranial nerve. Instillation of water into the external meatus is, of course, contraindicated for patients with perforation of the tympanic membrane due to middle ear disease. Table 6.5 shows that there were nine patients in our series with an absence of oculocephalic reflexes in the first 24 hours after admission, and death occurred in eight. Absence of oculovestibular reflexes was recorded in six patients and all died. The pupillary response has traditionally held pride of place in the neurological assessment of the unconscious patient. The reason for this is that third-nerve palsy frequently occurs as part of the clinical picture of an expanding intracranial mass lesion (such as haemorrhage) when the trunk of the nerve is compressed against the free edge of the tentorium because of herniation of the medial temporal lobe. In our experience pupillary changes in patients with intracranial haematoma generally only follow other signs of impairment of consciousness and the concern of medical and nursing staff with observation of the pupils in conscious patients is probably overemphasized. In the unconscious patient, on the other hand, the pupil reflex has great value as a measure of brain-stem function (Plum and Posner, 1976). A unilateral dilated pupil with no reaction to light may not only be due to a third-nerve palsy but also to optic nerve damage, and these two should be differentiated by the crossed responses. Bilateral lack of pupillary responses in unconscious patients suggests a poor prognosis. Within the first twenty-four hours of coma, ten of our patients had no pupillary response and six died (Table 6.5).

The corneal reflex is usually preserved after head injury except where patients are in deep coma; its absence suggests a poor prognosis. Nine of our cases had absent corneal reflexes during the first twenty-four hours after admission and seven died (Table 6.5).

A variety of other brain-stem responses may be seen in the unconscious head injury patient. Grimacing to pain is not uncommon and is usually associated with either a flexor or a localizing motor response. In patients in the early stages of the vegetative state, facial grimacing may develop before the motor response becomes flexor and, in some patients, facial grimacing without limb movement in response to pain may be a sign of spinal cord damage. Absence of the pharyngeal reflex is of practical importance as it indicates that the patient is unlikely to be able to cope with his own secretions and is in need of meticulous nursing care. Spontaneous coughing, swallowing and hiccupping in the unconscious patient are of little significance although their presence implies a grossly intact medulla. In some patients, for instance in a case already noted (229), the recovery of spontaneous coughing and swallowing is associated with the development of the vegetative state.

In general our experience of brain-stem responses in the Newcastle study was similar to that recorded in other centres (Jadhav et al, 1971; Poulsen and Zilstorff, 1972; Jennett et al, 1976). Absence of the brain-stem reflexes usually indicates a poor prognosis, but this is not an absolutely reliable predictor of outcome.

Autonomic Function

The practical importance of assessing respiration, pulse and blood pressure in unconscious patients needs no emphasis. A variety of abnormal respiratory patterns may be seen after head injury. Rapid regular respiration (Leigh and Shaw, 1976) may occur in patients with primary brain-stem injury and, as we have noted in Case 229, increase in respiration may occur as part of a tonic fit. Formal recording of respiratory patterns was not undertaken in our patients. However, in two instances (Cases 108 and 130) there were interesting changes in respiratory pattern associated with the development of cerebral oedema and decreasing level of consciousness. On admission both patients had periodic (Cheyne-Stokes) respiration and, as their consciousness level deteriorated, they developed irregular or ataxic respiration (Plum and Posner, 1976) as a prelude to complete cessation of spontaneous breathing. Both patients were treated vigorously in an attempt to reduce cerebral oedema and both were placed on ventilators but to no avail. At autopsy there was evidence in both cases of extensive hemisphere swelling with uncal and tentorial herniation.

The Cushing response — increasing blood pressure and falling pulse rate in association with rising intracranial pressure — is uncommon. Changes in pulse and blood pressure often indicate an injury elsewhere in the body although pulse increase is common in tonic spasms. High fever and excess sweating may be seen in association with decerebrate or tonic spasms and in patients with hypothalamic damage, though in practice secondary infection is more often the explanation. Excessive salivation, lacrimation and sebum secretion are all seen in patients in the vegetative state. Lacrimation in response to a painful stimulus is particularly common and often occurs in patients who are so deeply comatose that they are unlikely to 'feel' the pain.

Although not necessarily relevant to the assessment of coma, there are two aspects of the neurological examination of the acutely head injured patient that may conveniently be mentioned here: the observation of the optic fundus and the testing for signs of subarachnoid haemorrhage.

The Optic Fundus in Head Injury

Fundal abnormalities are common in the unconscious head-injured patient. Blot or flame-shaped haemorrhages may be seen and occasionally there may be frank subhyaloid haemorrhage. Ten of our patients had retinal haemorrhages and eight of them had suffered frontal head injuries. Papilloedema may develop within a few hours of a severe head injury and we have seen one such example. A lesser degree of papilloedema may develop within a few days of injury and then it is usually associated with traumatic subarachnoid haemorrhage. We have seen six such examples of papilloedema and in each case it resolved within a week or two.

Traumatic Subarachnoid Haemorrhage

If lumbar puncture were to be performed routinely after head injury, there would be blood-staining of the cerebrospinal fluid (c.s.f.) in a surprisingly high proportion of cases. Any head injury severe enough to produce cortical or meningeal contusion may cause slight bleeding into the subarachnoid space, but frank haemorrhage into the c.s.f. is seen only after severe injuries (i.e., those associated with a period of post-traumatic amnesia in excess of twelve hours).

In the Newcastle study, lumbar puncture was not performed routinely. Eighty-one of the patients were found to have a stiff neck within the first week of injury, but in many instances this was assumed to be the result of minor 'whiplash' injury to the cervical spine. Twenty-two patients were thought to have suffered a true traumatic subarachnoid haemorrhage. The common pattern of this syndrome is illustrated by the history of one of the patients in the study (Case 153).

The patient was a man of 35 who was injured as the result of an assault. On admission to hospital he was drowsy and confused and showed irritability; he resented examination and lay in bed curled up on his side. Attempts to talk to or examine him were met with abuse, but he was thought to have slight neck stiffness; lumbar puncture produced blood-stained c.s.f. Within 24 hours he became more alert; on the following day it was possible to hold a confused conversation with him and formal examination became feasible. He had no focal neurological signs but there was slight papilloedema with a flame-shaped haemorrhage in the right fundus. The papilloedema subsided within ten days of admission and the patient returned to normal. His period of post-traumatic amnesia was finally assessed at seven days.

SUMMARY

In this chapter we have considered some of the neurological signs that are often encountered in patients in coma as a result of head injury and we have referred to their value in relation to prognosis. The Glasgow head injury study (Jennett et al, 1976) has given careful consideration to the predictive value of the early physical signs and their pattern of change; our own observations are consistent with the Glasgow findings. In the following chapter we shall consider the neurological sequelae observed in patients after recovery from coma.

REFERENCES

Caveness, W. F. & Walker, A. E. (1966) *Head Injury.* Conference Proceedings. Philadelphia: J. H. Lippincott.

Jadhav, W. R., Sinha, A., Tandon, P. N., Kacker, S. K. & Banarji, A. K. (1971) Cold caloric test in altered states of consciousness. *The Laryngoscope,* **81,** 391-402.

Jennett, B. & Plum, F. (1972) Persistent vegetative state after brain damage. *Lancet,* **i,** 734-737.

Jennett, W. B., Teasdale, G., Braakman, R., Minderhoud, J. & Knill-Jones, R. (1976) Predicting outcome in individual patients after severe head injury. *Lancet,* **i,** 1031-1034.

Jennett, W. B., Teasdale, G., Braakman, R., Minderhoud, J., Heiden, J. & Kurze, T. (1979) Prognosis of patients with severe head injury. *Neurosurgery,* **4,** 283-289.

Leigh, R. J. & Shaw, D. A. (1976) Rapid regular respiration in unconscious patients. *Archives of Neurology,* **33,** 356-361.

Medical Research Council, Brain Injuries Committee (1941) A glossary of psychological terms commonly used in cases of head injury. *Medical Research Council War Memorandum No. 4.* London: Her Majesty's Stationery Office.

Ommaya, A. K. (1966) Trauma to the nervous system. *Annals of the Royal College of Surgeons of England,* **39,** 317-347.

Plum, F. & Posner, J. B. (1976) *The Diagnosis of Stupor and Coma.* Philadelphia: F. A. Davis.

Poulsen, J. & Zilstorff, K. (1972) Prognostic value of the caloric-vestibular test in the unconscious patient with cranial trauma. *Acta Neurological Scandinavica,* **48,** 282-292.

Symonds, C. P. (1937) Mental disorder following head injury. *Proceedings of the Royal Society of Medicine, London,* **30,** 1081-1083.

Teasdale, G. & Jennett, B. (1974) Assessment of impaired consciousness and coma: a practical scale. *Lancet,* **ii,** 81-84.

Teasdale, G., Galbraith, S. & Clarke, K. (1975) Acute impairment of brain function 2. Observation record chart. *Nursing Times,* **71,** 65-66.

Teasdale, G., Knill-Jones, R. & Van der Sand, J. (1978) Observer variability in assessing impaired consciousness and coma. *Journal of Neurology, Neurosurgery and Psychiatry,* **41,** 603-610.

CHAPTER SEVEN

The Neurological Sequelae of Head Injury

In this chapter we shall discuss the neurological complications and sequelae, other than coma, that may be encountered after head injury. They are many and varied, and disturbances of memory are among the most obvious. The amount of residual neurological damage in most cases of head injury bears some relation to the duration of coma, but in retrospect it is often extremely difficult for the clinician to determine its extent with any degree of accuracy. In this kind of circumstance an accurate assessment of memory loss may be of particular value in the overall evaluation of the head-injured patient. Memory disturbances of differing order and bearing different temporal relationships to the moment of injury are well recognized: the amnesia resulting from failure of registration during the period of unconsciousness, the amnesia for events leading up to the moment of loss of consciousness, and the amnesia that may follow recovery of consciousness that may considerably exceed the actual period of unconsciousness.

RETROGRADE AMNESIA

Retrograde amnesia is defined as partial or total loss of ability to recall events that have occurred during the period immediately preceding brain injury. Injury in this context embraces a wide variety of insults including epilepsy, electro-convulsive therapy, infections of the nervous system, high fever, anaesthesia, and, of course, concussion (Wolpaw, 1971). In the case of concussion, events that have occurred during the period of retrograde amnesia must often have been dramatic and registrable by a normal sensorium; yet the injury supervenes and memory of the events is not retained, or else it is retained but cannot be recalled. In many instances retrograde amnesia is only momentary, although in severe injury its duration is longer. Indeed, it was suggested by Russell and Nathan (1946) that there is a correlation between the severity of injury and the duration of retrograde amnesia, but this is now disputed.

A remarkable feature of the phenomenon of retrograde amnesia is its tendency to shrink during the period of recovery. While the patient is still confused the duration of retrograde amnesia may appear very long but, with improvement, it gradually diminishes. The period of post-traumatic amnesia (see below) invariably reaches its limits, indicating normal registration and recall of ongoing events, before retrograde amnesia shrinks to its final dimension. During the period of shrinkage isolated events may be recalled and so recovery is patchy. By the time retrograde amnesia has contracted to a few minutes, the patient's mental function is usually about normal. Occasionally retrograde amnesia may last for as long as a few days even when the patient has fully recovered, but it is extremely rare for it to exceed the period of post-traumatic amnesia (Russell and Nathan, 1946; Russell, 1971).

Numerous explanations for retrograde amnesia have been suggested. The most popular theory is that it is due to disturbance of short-term memory before it becomes encoded as long-term memory. Any satisfactory explanation must take account of the occurrence of prolonged retrograde amnesia and of the phenomenon of shrinkage. Wolpaw (1971) suggested that post-traumatic amnesia, by depriving pre-injury memories of a large proportion of their subsequent associations, might lead to retrograde amnesia; he thought that this theory would be compatible with the phenomenon of prolonged retrograde amnesia.

Wasterlain (1971) studied the pattern of retrograde amnesia in 47 patients with post-traumatic amnesia. In 20 of the cases the retrograde amnesia was of short duration and he suggested that in this group it was due to a failure of consolidation of memory. In the patients with prolonged periods of retrograde amnesia, Wasterlain found evidence of structural brain damage and he thought that in these cases the amnesia was due to failure of retrieval rather than of consolidation.

Interesting observations on retrograde amnesia were made by Yarnell and Lynch (1970) in a study of four patients immediately after brief concussion. One minute after the injury no retrograde amnesia could be demonstrated but, after an interval varying between ten and 30 minutes in the subjects studied, a period of retrograde amnesia could clearly be recognized. The explanation suggested was that continuing effects of concussive injury in the period following trauma may interfere with the fixation of short-term memory. It would be valuable if an opportunity arose to study further patients in this rather unique situation.

Retrograde amnesia cannot generally be shortened by barbiturate hypnosis, although exceptions to this rule have been recorded (Russell and Nathan, 1946). Occasionally, within a period of retrograde amnesia, there are islands of memory; by contrast, islands of memory loss located well outside the fixed period of retrograde amnesia may be detected in some patients (Williams and Zangwill, 1952).

The distribution of periods of retrograde amnesia in the Newcastle study is illustrated in Table 7.1. Figures are based on assessments made at the time of discharge from hospital and then at subsequent follow-up visits. There were 106 patients in whom the period of retrograde amnesia could not be assessed satisfactorily at the time of discharge; in many instances this was due to continuing confusion or dysphasia. Even at the late assessment, in 49 patients the duration of retrograde amnesia could not be determined. In some cases this was because of the severity of the neurological deficit, but this figure also includes a few patients who defaulted from follow-up visits. One patient at time of discharge appeared to have no retrograde amnesia, but at follow-up he could not recall events during the half minute or so prior to the injury. By contrast, in 15 patients there was good evidence of progressive shrinkage of the period of retrograde amnesia and the following are a few illustrative examples from their number.

Table 7.1. Duration of retrograde amnesia in patients on discharge and at follow-up (Newcastle study).

Period of retrograde amnesia	On discharge	Late assessment
Nil	64	63
Transient	154	186
< 1 minute	20	34
1—60 minutes	18	23
1—24 hours	9	13
1—7 days	1	4
> 7 days	0	0
Total assessable	*266*	*323*
Nonassessable	106	49
Total survivors	*372*	*372*

Case 92. This patient, a 51-year-old male admitted to hospital late one evening after a head injury, illustrates the possible influence of prompting on the recovery of retrograde amnesia. He had a bruise in the right occipital region but had no idea how it had occurred. He remembered starting the night-shift at about 6.00 p.m. but had no further recollection until his arrival in hospital. He had been seen at work at 8.30 p.m., when nothing amiss was noticed, but he was found an hour later wandering around his place of work in a state of confusion. While in hospital he was asymptomatic and no deficit was noted other than the period of amnesia. X-rays showed no evidence of skull fracture and he was discharged after a 24-hour period of observation.

When he was reviewed a month later, the patient was able to recount in some detail the events leading up to the injury. He had returned to work a week after the incident and encountered a mechanic who had been working with him on the evening in question. At this point events, as he put it, 'suddenly fell into place' and he remembered that he had been hit on the head by a falling block of wood. He could recall seeing the wood falling towards his head and putting up his hand to protect himself. He could not remember the actual impact and there was a blank in his memory until he found himself in the ambulance on the way to hospital. His final period of retrograde amnesia was in the 'transient' category, and post-traumatic amnesia was assessed at between half and one hour.

Case 10. This patient provides a further example of shrinking retrograde amnesia. He was a 16-year-old boy who was injured when he ran into the back of a stationary vehicle on his motorcycle. He suffered a fracture of the middle cranial fossa and on admission to hospital he was shocked and confused. He underwent immediate laparotomy for removal of a ruptured spleen and was still confused on recovery from the anaesthetic. He remained in this state for the first two days in hospital and claimed to have no recollection of events leading up to the accident or following it. By the fourth day, whilst he still could remember nothing prior to the accident, he was orientated in time and space and he could recall being examined on the previous evening. Twenty-four hours later he had a clear recollection of the events of the preceding 36 hours; his period of post-traumatic amnesia appeared fixed at four days. By this time he could remember some of the events that took place on the day before his accident and 24 hours later he could remember getting out of bed and dressing on the morning of the accident. At subsequent follow-up visits there was no further change in his recollection; the period of retrograde amnesia was fixed at thirty minutes and that of post-traumatic amnesia at four days.

There are obviously pitfalls in the assessment of memory defects in head injury and it would be a mistake to assume that the duration of retrograde amnesia can be recorded accurately in all cases. Nevertheless, there is a degree of consistency in the patterns that we encounter, and the calculated periods of retrograde amnesia are probably reliable in the majority of cases. In our own study, only 17 patients had a period of retrograde amnesia in excess of one hour and most of these had had severe head injuries with prolonged post-traumatic amnesia.

POST-TRAUMATIC AMNESIA

Post-traumatic amnesia may be defined as the time lapse between the accident and the point at which the functions concerned with memory are judged to have been restored. It is thus a retrospective determination which can only be made after the patient has recovered. Once day-to-day memory function has returned to normal, the period of post-traumatic amnesia may shrink.

Occasionally patients who suffer head injury recall clearly the details of their accident and the events immediately following it, but then later on enter a period of amnesia. About one in 40 closed head injuries is said to show this sequence of events, but Russell and Nathan (1946) have pointed out that the phenomenon is much commoner in gunshot wounds, where it occurs in about 14 per cent of cases. Presumably in these cases it is not the initial injury that disturbs consciousness and the mechanisms of memory, but the subsequent development of cerebral oedema. Fisher (1966) reported a patient with a closed head injury who developed post-traumatic amnesia without having suffered concussion or loss of consciousness.

Impairment of consciousness is not therefore a prerequisite for the extension of post-traumatic amnesia. Probably all that is disturbed during the extending period is the long-term registration of memory traces and at the time the patient may appear superficially to be perfectly normal. Because of this apparent normality, it is easy to underestimate the extent of post-traumatic amnesia and assume prematurely that it has terminated. Obliteration of memory throughout the period associated with post-traumatic amnesia is not uniformly complete. There may be islands of memory and these are usually concerned with special events such as the arrival of visitors. Such unevenness is only to be expected, bearing in mind the variable performance of memory in perfectly normal circumstances. Another odd feature is that patients may confabulate during the period of post-traumatic amnesia and this may well mislead the unskilled observer who assumes the patient to be normal.

One of the most striking things about post-traumatic amnesia in closed head injuries is that it correlates so well with the degree of severity (Russell, 1935; Russell and Nathan, 1946; Russell and Smith, 1961; Russell, 1971). Injuries resulting in post-traumatic amnesia of greater than 12 hours are generally classified as severe, and are associated with a high incidence of epilepsy or mental impairment, motor disorder or other organic residual deficit. One of the advantages of post-traumatic amnesia as a clinical measure is that it can be assessed in retrospect and it is probably the best available clinical indicator of head injury severity. However, it should be emphasized that the correlation does not hold good in either penetrating or crush injuries, where severe damage may occur in the absence of impairment of consciousness or a recognizable period of post-traumatic amnesia. One other point of note is that the duration of post-traumatic amnesia after injuries of comparable severity tends to increase with advancing age and it is a well-recognized fact that elderly people fare less well after head injury than do the young.

Our observations on post-traumatic amnesia in the Newcastle series are summarized in Table 7.2. It is based on assessments made both on discharge and at follow-up

Table 7.2. Duration of post-traumatic amnesia in patients on discharge and at follow-up (Newcastle study).

Period of post-traumatic amnesia	On discharge	Late assessment
Nil	38	38
< 1 minute	24	21
1—5 minutes	39	39
5—15 minutes	17	17
15—60 minutes	68	70
1—6 hours	43	44
6—12 hours	11	12
12—24 hours	17	18
1—7 days	16	37
>7 days	1	34
Total	*274*	*330*
Unknown	32	42
'Extending'	66	0
Total survivors	*372*	*372*

interview. Fifty-six per cent of the patients in whom a final assessment could be made had post-traumatic amnesia lasting for less than an hour, and in 73 per cent the period was less than 12 hours. In 66 patients post-traumatic amnesia was still thought to be extending at the time of discharge from hospital; in 32 patients no satisfactory assessment could be made. A final assessment of post-traumatic amnesia was made in 330 patients and it was not adequately assessable in 42. A correlation between the duration of post-traumatic amnesia and the initial level of consciousness on admission is illustrated in Table 7.3, which provides some support for the view that post-traumatic amnesia is a measure of head injury severity. By contrast, our figures do not suggest that there is any particular relationship between the duration of post-traumatic amnesia and the presence or absence of skull fracture (Table 7.4). No fewer than 17 patients with no detectable post-traumatic amnesia in fact had skull fractures, and it is generally recognized that their presence or absence is not a good guide to the severity of the head injury.

Table 7.3. Post-traumatic amnesia and conscious level (Ommaya Scale — Table 6.1) on admission to hospital (Newcastle series).

Period of post-traumatic amnesia	Ommaya Scale					Total
	1	2	3	4	5	
Zero	38	0	0	0	0	38
Transient	21	0	0	0	0	21
>5 minutes	39	0	0	0	0	39
5—15 minutes	17	0	0	0	0	17
15—60 minutes	68	2	0	0	0	70
2—6 hours	42	2	0	0	0	44
6—12 hours	7	5	0	0	0	12
12—24 hours	7	11	0	0	0	18
1—7 days	0	33	4	0	0	37
>7 days	0	24	9	1	0	34
Not known	33	4	5	0	0	42
Total survivors	*272*	*81*	*18*	*1*	*0*	*372*

Table 7.4. Post-traumatic amnesia and skull fracture (Newcastle series).

Period of post-traumatic amnesia	No fracture	Fracture	No X-ray	Total
Nil	21	17		38
<1 minute	14	7		21
1—5 minutes	34	5		39
6—15 minutes	12	5		17
6—60 minutes	66	4		70
1—6 hours	42	1	1	44
7—12 hours	8	4		12
13—24 hours	10	8		18
1—7 days	19	18		37
>7 days	14	11	9	34
Not known	34	8		42
Total survivors	*274*	*88*	*10*	*372*

PERSISTING MEMORY IMPAIRMENT

Before leaving the subject of memory we should recall that, apart from the specific syndromes discussed above, a number of patients have continuing disorders of memory as a result of severe head injury. The severity of these memory defects has been shown by Brooks (1976) to be related to the length of post-traumatic amnesia, and the relationship is particularly significant in older patients. Persisting memory defects, impairment of intellectual function, and global dementia may all be encountered as after-effects of severe head injury, but these will be discussed later when we are considering the psychiatric sequelae.

SYNDROMES ATTRIBUTABLE TO FOCAL BRAIN INJURY

Thus far we have been discussing syndromes that result from the 'generalized' effects of a closed head injury. We will now consider a number of neural functions which may be impaired singly or in combination; damage, when it does occur, is presumed to be due to focal brain injury such as contusion, laceration or tearing of fibre tracts as a result of shearing strain (Strich, 1969). Generally speaking, the lesions about to be discussed occur most frequently in the context of moderate or severe generalized brain injury. They are, therefore, associated in the majority of instances with post-traumatic amnesias in excess of 12 hours. The obvious exception is focal brain damage occurring as a result of a penetrating injury, which may have minimal general effects. In the following paragraphs a variety of the more commonly encountered focal deficits resulting from head injury will be considered.

Defects of Motor Function after Head Injury

It is generally believed — and there is a certain amount of supporting evidence (Miller and Stern, 1965; Fahy, Irving and Millac, 1967) — that hemiplegia and other motor deficits resulting from head injury carry a good prognosis. The data upon which these assumptions are made are fairly limited and there are few studies in which serial improvement in motor function after head injury is documented. In the study of Miller and Stern (1965) 25 patients with motor weakness resulting from head injury were re-examined after a mean interval of 11 years. All were thought to have improved and only four were found to have any residual weakness. Even when gait disturbance after head injury is due to both cerebellar and pyramidal involvement, the prognosis is still thought to be good. However, Walker and Erculei (1969) have made the comment that patients with residual motor deficit are particularly liable to develop post-traumatic epilepsy.

In the Newcastle series 55 patients out of the total of 372 had a hemiparesis at the time of discharge from hospital. In 30 patients the right limbs were involved and in 25 the left. The hemiparesis was graded as 'mild' in 39 patients and as 'severe' in 16. As is shown in Table 7.5, there had been considerable improvement by the time of the two-year follow-up. Of the 16 patients who initially had a severe hemiparesis, there were only two with a similar degree of deficit after two years; five had improved but had a residual mild deficit whereas nine had recovered function completely, although in some there was still reflex asymmetry. Among the 39 patients whose hemiparesis was initially graded as 'mild', 16 were left with persisting deficit, 21 recovered completely by the end of two years and two were lost to follow-up. All those who suffered a hemiparesis in our series had a period of post-traumatic amnesia of more than 24 hours. In general, our figures would seem to confirm previous observations on the relatively good prognosis for recovery of motor deficits after head injury.

Table 7.5. Patients with hemiparesis on discharge and at two-year follow-up (Newcastle series).

	At discharge	At 2-year follow-up
Hemiparesis		
mild	39	21
severe	16	2
Lost to follow-up	0	2
Recovered	0	30
Total	55	55

Occipital Lobe Injuries

A substantial literature has accumulated on the subject of visual disorders resulting from head injuries involving the occipital lobes. Strauss and Savitsky (1934) described in detail the various types of field defect they had encountered. Symonds (1960) was interested in this, as in other aspects of head injury, and he drew particular attention to the rarity of visual agnosia as a manifestation of trauma. In more recent times, Gjerris (1976) has reviewed the subject of visual disorder after head injury and has discussed the defects that may result from lesions at various points in the visual pathways.

There has been particular interest in the visual disturbances that are sometimes encountered in children after head injury. Bodian (1964) described the occurrence of transient blindness after relatively mild injuries in childhood; subsequent studies have suggested that in the majority of cases the disturbance has originated in the occipital lobes (Griffith and Dodge, 1968; Weisz, Hemli and Kraus, 1975). In these cases vision usually recovers and it is suggested that the disorder may be due to temporary occipital lobe ischaemia induced by vasospasm.

In our own series the number of patients with visual-field defects resulting from postchiasmatic lesions was small; indeed there were only three. Two of them had depressed fractures in the occipital region and both were seen to have cortical lacerations at operation. In neither case did the visual-field defect recover. The third patient had a closed injury associated with a traumatic subarachnoid haemorrhage. Although he was confused when he was admitted to hospital, a homonymous hemianopia was demonstrable and it was still present two days later when he was transferred to his local hospital. It was subsequently reported to have improved but, unfortunately, detailed follow-up information was not available because the patient died suddenly a month after the accident as a result of a myocardial infarct.

Parietal Lobe Injuries

We encountered no specific examples of parietal lobe disturbance in our series although they are described in the context of head injury. Cortical sensory loss can occur but it is rarely incapacitating and usually has a good prognosis. Specific disorders such as agnosia and apraxia are probably uncommon, but it is possible that their recognition is obscured by other more obvious defects of higher function resulting from the injury. Strauss and Savitsky (1934) drew particular attention to the occurrence of alexia resulting from injury, which in their cases was commonly associated with right homonymous hemianopia. As in the case of other cortical disturbances, patients with parietal lobe lesions as a result of head injury have an increased incidence of epilepsy.

Speech disorders after Head Injury

Disorders both of language and of articulation are encountered as a result of head injury (Wallace, 1969).

Aphasia

The problem of aphasia following head injury has been extensively studied, particularly in patients who have suffered penetrating injuries in war (Russell and Espir, 1961). In civilian practice the majority of injuries are of the closed variety and a much smaller proportion result in aphasia. In a study of 255 patients with head injury, Glaser and Shafer (1932) found that 16 (6 per cent) had aphasia. A smaller incidence was reported by Arseni and colleagues (1970) from Bucharest; they found 34 cases of aphasia among a total of 1544 head-injured patients, giving an incidence of 2.2 per cent. This figure is near to the 2 per cent incidence reported by Heilman, Safran and Geschwind (1971) from Boston on the basis of a study of approximately 750 patients with closed head injury. By and large, patients in this category have a good prognosis. On the other hand, Heilman, Safran and Geschwind (1971) emphasized in their prospective study that the prognosis was variable. The majority of their patients had an anomic aphasia but there were often other associated defects of higher cortical function which might militate against a good recovery. Furthermore they had some problems with follow-up which they recognized might lead to their underestimating the degree of recovery of some patients. They were unable to identify any particular features that helped them to predict outcome in their aphasic patients.

In the more recent study of Levine, Grossman and Kelly (1976) 50 patients, most of whom had severe head injuries, were studied in detail with a variety of refined aphasia tests. On the basis of these tests, naming and word-finding defects were found in almost half the patients. Twenty-one were said to have an aphasic disorder of one sort or another. The authors emphasized that it is in the severe closed injury that aphasia is encountered and thus there is usually evidence of lengthy post-traumatic amnesia.

Returning to the question of prognosis, Wallace (1969) has emphasized the importance of speech therapy and described in detail her experience of treating 29 patients between the ages of five and 25 years. The majority had improved within six to nine months of the date of injury. Thomsen (1975) studied twelve aphasic patients from a group of 26 with severe closed head injuries and showing unconsciousness of more than 24 hours duration. In all except one, there was good recovery of aphasia.

Dysarthria

In patients with disturbances of articulation after head injury, there is usually other evidence of brain damage. There is not much information on overall incidence but Wallace (1969) describes 13 cases of dysarthria among 363 patients with severe injury. Hermann (1965) also emphasizes the severity of injury when considering dysarthria and comments on the fact that it is often part of a generalized cerebellar disturbance. In her patients, the majority of injuries had produced extensive brain-stem damage with prolonged coma, and the residual dysarthria was associated with severe disorders of gait. The majority of her cases showed significant improvement although there was usually some residual clumsiness. She identifies three subgroups within her group of patients with dysarthria after head injury:

1. Patients whose dysarthria was predominantly cerebellar in type. In her experience they showed the greatest degree of spontaneous improvement, and speech tended to recover before the other motor disabilities.
2. This group is in striking contrast to the first. The patients had a combined pyramidal and extra-pyramidal disorder, and speech was of poor volume and monotonous pitch; it had the disturbed rhythm that is characteristic of extrapyramidal disorder. In these patients, speech showed little sign of improvement and remained a major difficulty, in contrast to the other motor signs which improved to a remarkable degree.
3. Patients in the third group were suffering essentially from spastic dysarthrias. Their prognosis was good and the view was expressed that it is this group that is likely to obtain most benefit from speech therapy.

Finally, there is the rare occurrence of articulatory difficulty in patients who suffer lower cranial nerve palsies as a result of basal skull fractures. The prognosis of these is said to be good.

The Newcastle series — speech disorders

Twenty-five patients in the Newcastle series had speech defects at the time of their discharge from hospital. One was dysphonic but this was attributed to trauma to the vocal cords during intubation in the Emergency Department. The dysphonia persisted for a week and then recovered completely.

Dysarthria was recorded in seven patients but in only one was it severe in degree (Case 193):

This was a man of 20 who was injured when the car he was driving was involved in a collision. There was no sign of external injury and no skull fracture. He was comatose for four days after admission; he did not open his eyes or vocalize, but he showed spontaneous limb movements and a localizing motor response to pain. On the fifth day he began to open his eyes and obey simple commands if they were issued with sufficient vigour. Nevertheless, there was no indication that he could vocalize and he uttered only occasional meaningless sounds. By the eleventh day he could sit up in bed and take notice but still could not produce any intelligible words. His tendon reflexes were brisk and his plantar responses were extensor. Gradually over the next few days he developed the ability to communicate but it became apparent that he had a profound dysarthria. It had a combination of spastic and ataxic elements and the accompanying difficulty in his walking had the same motor characteristics. Two years after the accident he still had mild dysarthria and minimal residual ataxia of gait. There were no signs of spasticity except that his tendon reflexes remained brisk. This patient had a period of post-traumatic amnesia that was estimated at four to six weeks.

We have already drawn attention to the anomalous failure of speech in contrast to a reasonably high score in the other responses in the Coma Scale, and have indicated that it should alert us to the possibility of a primary abnormality of speech. In our experience this has usually been an aphasia, but the speech defect in the case described above was purely dysarthric.

Seventeen of our patients were aphasic during their initial stay in hospital. All had suffered severe closed injuries and all were right-handed. Ten of them also had a right hemiparesis. The following cases illustrate the potential for recovery even after severe dysphasia.

Case 380. A lady of 55 had a road accident while driving. She suffered a right-frontal head injury, and an underlying fracture was demonstrated. On admission, there was no response to vocal commands and no eye-opening to pain, but a painful stimulus elicited localizing responses in the upper limbs. Within six hours of admission she opened her eyes and began to obey simple commands. In response to being questioned she would simply repeat a single word and obviously she had marked verbal perseveration. Within 24 hours she was alert but there was evidence of weakness of the right arm and a profound aphasia. She needed great encouragement to attempt any spontaneous speech and she showed marked paraphasic substitutions. Comprehension of anything more than single-order commands was severely impaired and she had difficulty in repeating even single words. After a further 24 hours she had improved markedly and by the time two weeks had elapsed from the date of injury, speech had improved to the extent that she could hold a rational conversation; the only defect was slight hesitancy and an occasional naming difficulty. At the six-month follow-up, speech was recorded as normal. In this case the period of post-traumatic amnesia had been assessed as seven days.

Case 254. This was an 18-year-old male who was injured when the car he was driving was involved in a road accident. He had a single major convulsion shortly after admission to hospital and by the time 12 hours had elapsed he showed the typical picture of traumatic subarachnoid haemorrhage with headache, restlessness, neck stiffness and irritability provoked by any attempt at formal examination. Such interference resulted in groaning, but he did not produce any recognizable words. All tendon reflexes, including the jaw jerk, were pathologically brisk and the right plantar response was extensor. Over the next few days he became increasingly noisy and aggressive; he moaned incessantly but still did not produce any recognizable language. By the fourth day he was less noisy and would open his eyes occasionally and obey simple commands. At this stage it was noted that he had mild bilateral papilloedema.

By the end of two weeks he was answering simple questions but only with repeated prompting. With subsequent improvement it became obvious that he had a definite speech defect and he tended to repeat questions and to perseverate. Tests of comprehension suggested severe impairment. Nevertheless, he continued to improve over the next few weeks and finally went home eight weeks after the accident. By this time he was able to converse fluently in spite of occasional paraphasic errors. The tendon reflexes remained brisk and the right plantar response was still extensor. In addition to the speech defect, intellectual impairment was suspected; on the Weschler Adult Intelligence Scale his verbal IQ was measured at 130, with a performance level of 111. Fifteen months after the accident he obtained three satisfactory GCE 'A' level passes and entered university.

This boy was regarded as having had a severe head injury, and the period of post-traumatic amnesia was estimated at six weeks. The striking thing about his case was the remarkable degree of improvement in relation to both his aphasia and his undoubted intellectual impairment.

All our patients with dysphasia showed considerable improvement and 15 were ultimately thought to be back to normal at two-year follow-up. One patient had a mild residual naming defect and we failed to obtain follow-up information on another. It should be emphasized that there were no penetrating injuries in the left hemisphere in our cohort.

Other Focal Cerebral Syndromes

In addition to the relatively common focal sequelae that we have been considering, there are a number of reports in the literature of interesting and unusual syndromes, most of which have been identified as a result of sophisticated neuropsychological testing. We will not attempt a comprehensive essay into this fascinating and highly specialized field whose boundaries will doubtless extend in the future. However, one or two examples may be cited. Humphrey and Zangwill (1951) described three patients in whom there was a dramatic cessation of dreaming as a result of head injury. All of them were aware of difficulty with visual memory while they were awake. One of the patients eventually started having dreams again but this was not so in the other two cases. Newcombe et al (1971) have described defects in recognition in patients with focal brain injuries, and Yin (1970) has studied the specific problem of inability to recognize faces in similarly affected patients.

LATE EFFECTS OF SEVERE BRAIN INJURY

At the beginning of the last chapter we gave a broad outline of the types of head injury commonly encountered, with arbitrary grading into four categories according to the degree of severity. We referred to the fact that patients in the most severe grade showed features of 'primary brain-stem injury', which so often has a fatal outcome. The pathological findings in such fatal cases have been well documented (Crompton, Teare and Bowen, 1966; Jellinger and Seitelberger, 1970; Crompton, 1971). Whilst the concept of primary brain-stem injury is useful clinically, the pathological evidence points to the fact that it is only a part of diffuse brain damage (Mitchell and Adams, 1973). Some patients do survive after these very severe injuries (Kremer, Russell and Smythe, 1947), and Jooma (1972) has even suggested that in the early stages these survivors have a characteristic EEG pattern. The fact that survival can possible occur even after secondary brain-stem haemorrhage is also relevant to a discussion of the late effects of such injuries (Caplan and Zervas, 1977).

A wide range of neurological deficits may be encountered in these survivors of severe injury. Bricolo (1976) has written an excellent review of the neurological sequelae in patients who have suffered prolonged post-traumatic coma. Such patients are likely to have shown decerebrate rigidity and tonic fits at an early stage after injury, and the survivors are almost invariably left with gross impairment of intellectual function. A variety of motor deficits may result from these injuries and there may be a mixture of cerebellar, pyramidal and striatal signs. Patients not infrequently show bilateral pyramidal signs accompanied by severe rigidity, but a true Parkinsonian syndrome is rarely seen. Involuntary movements such as chorea, tremor or myoclonus are likewise rare. On the other hand, dystonic posturing of the limbs with pseudo-bulbar dysarthria, dysphagia and emotional lability are relatively common. Cerebellar signs are infrequently encountered and when they do occur they are attributable either to direct laceration of cerebellar hemispheres, or to tearing of cerebellar tracts as a result of shearing strains. Generally speaking, cerebellar signs following severe head injury have a good prognosis for recovery (Arne, 1975).

One of the patients in the Newcastle series had a very striking disorder of movement following his severe head injury. He was a boy of 15 who had a severe head injury as a result of a road accident and, on admission to hospital, he had the typical signs of primary brain-stem damage. He made a gradual recovery and, after an interval of three months, was able to take a few steps, but had marked spasticity and profound dysarthria. At that stage he had a very slight Parkinsonian-type tremor of the left hand. By six months he was able to walk and speak reasonably well but the tremor of the left hand had become very marked; it was increased by action with terminal accentuation and he was quite incapacitated by it. Eventually the tremor showed all the features of a dentato-rubral lesion and it became associated with severe titubation.

We have referred previously to the disturbances of eye movements that are seen in the acute stages of these severe injuries. It is uncommon for supranuclear or internuclear ophthalmoplegias to persist, and skew deviations and nystagmus also tend to recover.

The type of head injury we are now considering is a particularly gloomy one. As already stated, a high proportion die and those that recover are likely to suffer the severe disabilities that we have just been describing. But perhaps the worst feature of all is that some patients survive but remain insentient — awake but unaware. They require total nursing care and their pitiable condition causes much sorrow for their families.

The Persistent Vegetative State

This term was introduced by Jennett and Plum (1972) to describe the condition of these hapless survivors. The syndrome in question has previously been referred to as the apallic state or as akinetic mutism. Perhaps more correctly, it has also been referred to as akinetic mutism with spastic tetraplegia.

In the patients we are talking about, the injury has always been severe and decerebrate rigidity and abnormalities of brain-stem function are invariably present from the early stages of coma. Such patients 'recover' to the extent that they develop spontaneous eye-opening and occasionally may appear to make following eye movements. But they do not speak or show more than minimal spontaneous motor activity, neither do they respond to verbal stimulation. Patients who show these features of the 'vegetative state' have a poor prognosis in terms of recovery but they may show prolonged survival (Jennett and Plum, 1972). With advances in methods of resuscitation and with technological improvements in life support equipment, there is an increasing risk that patients will be rescued from the initial dangers of catastrophic injuries only to be doomed to a type of survival that no one would wish for himself or for a member of his family. Considerations of this sort have led to some heart-searching over the question of early resuscitation and, more constructively, to attempts to develop accurate methods of predicting the likely outcome after severe head injury. As previously mentioned, Jennett and his colleagues in Glasgow are pioneers in the development and validation of methods of predicting outcome in the early stages. Both in the overall management of patients and in planning their rehabilitation programme, it would help to be able to predict also the final degree of recovery of those severely disabled, but conscious, patients who have survived the acute stage of their injury. Resources in rehabilitation would be most effectively used if they could be directed to those patients who have the greatest potential for recovery and re-establishment of an independent existence. The Glasgow studies have started to provide some information along these lines. They have shown that few of the patients still in the vegetative state one month after their injury will show significant improvement. A small proportion may show signs of recovery, but it is unlikely that any will ever regain an independent existence (Jennett, 1976).

In this chapter we have been concerned so far with sequelae in patients who have suffered severe injuries, but in the following paragraphs, dealing with cranial nerve deficits, we are concerned with patients whose head injuries may have been relatively minor.

CRANIAL NERVE INJURIES

At least ten per cent of all head injuries are complicated by damage to one or more cranial nerves. The site of the injury is crucial in determining which nerve may be affected. Those nerves issuing from the posterior fossa are in a protected situation and are rarely injured in isolation. Others may be damaged as a result of basal skull fractures. The third and sixth nerves are particularly vulnerable to intracranial shifts resulting from raised pressure. Details of cranial nerve defects due to head injury have been extensively reviewed (Russell, 1932; Strauss and Savitsky, 1934; Merritt, 1943; Brock, 1960; Rowbotham, 1964; Feiring, 1974; Vinken and Bruyn, 1976).

The Olfactory Nerve

Hughlings Jackson (1864) provided an early and probably original description of anosmia due to head injury. Indeed head injury is regarded as the most common cause of permanent anosmia (Schneider, 1972). The loss of smell is often bilateral and it is said to occur in from three to ten per cent of head injuries (Leigh, 1943; Sumner, 1964; Hagan, 1967; Mealey, 1968). Anosmia is thus one of the most common neurological deficits to follow head injury.

The myelinated fibres of the olfactory nerve have no capacity for regeneration. In some instances there is recovery of the sense of smell after a head injury; in such cases it is assumed that interruption of the olfactory pathways was incomplete. If recovery does take place, it is likely to do so within six months (Leigh, 1943; Sumner, 1964).

Anosmia is usually the result of a severe injury although it can occur after minor or even trivial trauma. The exact site of injury is important — frontal and occipital injuries have the highest incidence of anosmia (Goland, 1937; Sumner, 1964). Partial loss of smell after head injury is said to be quite common, but it is less likely to be recognized. There has recently been interest in the relationship between abnormalities of taste and smell and the levels of zinc in the blood and tissues. Schechter and Henkin (1974) have suggested that zinc levels are lower than normal in the serum of patients with post-traumatic disturbances of taste and smell.

As a rule, and for obvious reasons, anosmic patients have a disturbance in ability to taste; that is, to appreciate flavours. They frequently describe their need to add excessive amounts of salt or sauce to make food palatable. Occasionally, head-injured patients appear to lose their true sense of taste in addition to their sense of smell, and Sumner (1964) has suggested that the lesion in such cases may be central rather than peripheral.

Perversion of taste and smell may accompany anosmia after head injury, although this is a rare occurrence (Leigh, 1943; Sumner, 1964). Such perversions may occur spontaneously or following an olfactory stimulus and may result in food becoming quite unpleasant for the victim. Apart from causing deprivation of enjoyment of food, anosmia can also threaten a patient's safety, as in the case of a fire outbreak or a leakage of gas. Miller and Stern (1965) reported a patient who died from accidental coal-gas poisoning as a result of complete anosmia. The subject of post-traumatic anosmia and ageusia has been fully reviewed by Sumner (1976).

Bilateral anosmia was noted in 37 patients in the Newcastle series. Nine were female and 28 male; their ages ranged from 16 to 76 years. All had received injuries to the face or to the frontal or occipital region of the skull. Eighteen patients had skull fractures. The period of post-traumatic amnesia varied from nil in three cases to over a week in four. Taste was impaired in eight patients, and perversions of smell and taste (parosmia and parageusia) were noted in three. Seventeen patients in the series experienced some degree of recovery, always within six months of the injury. Those who recovered quickly had almost invariably suffered from swelling about the face and nose when the anosmia was first recorded, and several had bleeding noses. It seems likely, therefore, that the anosmia in a proportion of patients was due to local injury, without necessarily any involvement of the olfactory nerves. Anosmia in seven patients was accompanied by cerebrospinal fluid rhinorrhoea, and two patients in the series had suffered damage to the optic pathways. One patient with anosmia had a temporal bone fracture resulting in positional vertigo, impairment of hearing and a delayed facial palsy. Finally, there was one patient who clearly was simulating. He claimed to be unaware of a strong whiff of ammonia although his protestations were accompanied by severe lacrimation.

Disorders of the Optic Nerve

Blurring of vision is exceedingly common after head injury. Indeed, it was suggested by Russell (1932) that visual acuity is probably diminished temporarily in all severe head injuries. Pathological studies of fatal cases certainly show a high percentage with changes in the optic nerve and chiasm (Crompton, 1970). Often, however, the complaint of blurred vision after head injury is due to the development of awareness of pre-existing presbyopia or other refractive abnormality, in the rather anxious and introspective period of early recovery.

The literature on visual impairment after head injury has been reviewed by Gjerris (1976). A fairly wide incidence range of optic nerve damage has been quoted, but the figure of 1.5 per cent arrived at by Turner (1943) is probably about average. In closed injuries the optic nerve is most commonly damaged by blows in the frontal region, though often there is no fracture to be seen on x-ray. In the majority of cases the nerve is injured in the optic canal, and visual loss is immediate, although it should be noted that in some instances the blow to the head may have been quite mild. Recovery may occur within the first few days after injury but no improvement can be anticipated after the lapse of a month. Whilst direct damage to the optic nerve is the most common cause of visual impairment, interference with its blood supply is sometimes the mechanism of sight loss (Cullen, 1964; Wyllie, McLeod and Cullen, 1972). Hughes (1962) has discussed the various mechanisms whereby visual loss after head injury may be produced. Even in the early stages after injury when the patient is still unconscious, the absence of a pupillary light reflex may provide a clue to the presence of an optic nerve lesion. Optic atrophy after a traumatic nerve lesion takes up to four weeks to develop.

Injuries to the optic chiasm are rare and are only seen in severe injuries where classically the chiasm suffers a complete longitudinal tear (Traquair, Dott and Russell, 1935; Turner, 1943). Permanent field defects resulting from such lesions are rarely encountered because of the high mortality associated with the type of injury that causes them. Late visual impairment after head injury is uncommon, but the syndrome of post-traumatic chiasmatic arachnoiditis which sometimes produces it has been described (Fisher, 1965).

In the Newcastle series there were seven patients who had optic nerve or chiasm injuries (Table 7.6). Five of these had complete optic nerve lesions: two were associated with bilateral anosmia, one with a blow-out orbital fracture and two were isolated lesions. Of the remaining two patients, one had a partial optic nerve lesion in association with a severe head injury, and the final case (Case 407) was assumed to have a chiasmal lesion. This patient developed diabetes insipidus and persisting

Table 7.6. Optic nerve and chiasmal defects (Newcastle series).

Case no.	Age	Sex	Site	Fracture	Post-traumatic amnesia	Side	Other injuries	Outcome
82	63	M	R. frontal	R. frontal	0	R	Anosmia	Complete lesion; no recovery
87	57	M	R. eyelid	Nil	5 minutes	R	Nil	Complete lesion; no recovery
123	22	M	Face	Facial bones	10 days	L	Infraorbital blow-out fracture	Complete lesion; no recovery
248	46	M	L. frontal	L. frontal	8 hours	L	Positional nystagmus & vertigo	Complete lesion; no recovery
230	45	M	R. temporal	Nil	10 days	R	Positional nystagmus & vertigo	R. partial lesion; slight improvement
329	37	M	L. frontal	L. frontal	20 minutes	L	Anosmia. Diabetes insipidus	Complete lesion; no recovery
407	17	M	Bifrontal	Frontal	1 week	Bilateral	Diabetes insipidus Anosmia CSF rhinorrhoea	Right partial lesion; slight improvement. Left complete lesion; no recovery.

cerebrospinal fluid rhinorrhoea after a severe injury which had produced a period of post-traumatic amnesia of seven days. He had complete blindness in the left eye and a permanent temporal field deficit in the right. Three months after injury the diabetes insipidus had resolved, and detailed endocrine tests showed no demonstrable hypothalamic abnormality.

Disorders of Eye Movement (Third, Fourth and Sixth Cranial Nerves)

In the previous chapter, dealing with the acute neurological effects of head injury, we discussed the disturbances of eye movement that may be seen in head injury coma and in patients with primary brain-stem injury. Let us now consider the other abnormalities of eye movement that may be encountered as a sequel to head injury.

Persisting disorders due to central damage, other than in the context of coma, are extremely uncommon and are only seen after the most severe injuries. Keane (1975) analysed 100 cases of skew deviation of the eyes and attributed five of them to blunt head injury. He did not record for how long the skew deviation persisted. Other central abnormalities are equally uncommon and they rarely produce symptoms.

Diplopia after head injury is common and perhaps its most frequent cause is the breakdown of a previously asymptomatic phoria (Hart, 1969). In such cases, there is no evidence of any direct effect of head injury and it is more likely that it acts as a precipitant, as may fatigue, alcohol or general medical illness in those with a latent phoria.

Damage to the third, fourth or sixth nerve occurs in three to seven per cent of head injuries (Russell, 1960; Hughes, 1954). The third and sixth nerves are equally liable to injury whereas isolated damage to the fourth is uncommon. Despite this, a third of a particular series of 33 cases of isolated fourth nerve paresis were said to have been caused by trauma (Burger, Kalvin and Lawton-Smith, 1970). In general it is uncommon to see an eye movement abnormality after a minor head injury, though there is a case recorded of a patient who developed bilateral sixth nerve palsies following a minor injury in the absence of a skull fracture (Roberts and Owens, 1972). The prognosis for extraocular muscle paresis is good and the recovery rate is as high as 75 per cent.

Although head trauma seldom causes direct damage to the fourth cranial nerve, it may be associated with orbital injury, which can produce impairment of function of the superior oblique muscle. The so-called 'blow-out fracture' is often the main feature of these orbital injuries. Chapman et al (1970) have recorded six cases of bilateral superior oblique palsy due to trauma.

Persisting nystagmus is exceedingly uncommon after head injury. When nystagmus is seen, it is nearly always of the intermittent positional variety that is so commonly associated with post-traumatic dizziness (Chapter Ten). Occasionally there is persisting nystagmus and one example, quoted by Sabin and Poche (1969), describes a patient who appeared to develop rotational nystagmus as a result of a head injury. In addition to the nystagmus, this patient had a post-traumatic bitemporal hemianopia.

In the Newcastle series there were three patients who had third-nerve palsies, two as a result of direct injury and one as a result of an extradural haematoma which caused shift — a classical false localizing sign. In the latter case the third-nerve palsy recovered completely within 24 hours, whilst the palsies due to direct injury took much longer to recover. One was still apparent, although mild in degree, some two years after injury. Two of our patients had sixth-nerve palsies and in both instances recovery was complete. None of our patients had isolated fourth-nerve lesions, although three patients were thought to have evidence of superior oblique paresis as a result of direct injury to the orbit.

There were five other patients with persisting diplopia which was thought to be due entirely to orbital fracture. In three the diplopia was still present at the two-year follow-up. Six of our patients had diplopia at follow-up visits, which we attributed to the breaking down of a latent squint. The diplopia had not been present while they had been in hospital but had occurred subsequently. Five of these patients were poly-symptomatic and the majority of them were depressed. As other symptoms subsided, the double vision tended to resolve and only one patient required orthoptic exercises.

Trigeminal Nerve Injuries

The most vulnerable part of the trigeminal nerve is its supraorbital branch, which is often damaged by frontal laceration or by fracture of the upper margin of the orbit. There were eight supraorbital nerve lesions in our series. As a rule, the injury is of little significance and the sensory symptoms diminish with the passage of time. Nevertheless some patients do make rather heavy weather of the numbness, particularly in the medico-legal setting; others complain of persisting hyperaesthesia in the distribution of the nerve, sometimes associated with tenderness in any scarring that may be present. The infraorbital nerve is less often affected, but it may be damaged in patients with severe facial injuries. Our series included three patients with infraorbital nerve lesions resulting from facial fractures; one of these was a blow-out fracture of the orbit. As in the case of the supraorbital nerve, the sensory loss of infraorbital lesions is rarely disabling.

Occasionally a jaw fracture may result in damage to the inferior dental nerve. One unfortunate young lady in our series suffered such a lesion. She regarded the sensory impairment as a major disability as it diminished her enjoyment of kissing.

Damage to the intracranial portion of the trigeminal nerve is exceedingly uncommon as it is well protected in its course from the brain stem to Meckel's cave. It can be affected in particularly severe injuries with basal skull fractures, but we encountered no such lesions in the 404 patients in our study.

Facial Nerve Injuries

Facial paralysis is a relatively common sequel of head injury, occurring in approximately three per cent of cases (Russell, 1960). It usually results from a fracture of the petrous part of the temporal bone, though occasionally the nerve is damaged as it emerges from the stylomastoid foramen (Mealey, 1968). In about 50 per cent of patients with facial nerve palsy due to head injury there is concomitant evidence of damage to the structures of the middle and inner ear and bleeding from the external auditory meatus is common. Looking at it the other way around, 20 per cent of patients who bleed from an ear after head injury have an ipsilateral facial palsy (Russell, 1960). Bilateral facial nerve paralysis is rare and usually occurs in patients with extensive basal fractures or with crush injuries of the skull.

Turner (1944) studied 70 patients with facial nerve palsy following head injury. They fell into two roughly equal groups. In 36 patients the facial palsy followed immediately after the injury and 27 of them made a good recovery. Thirty-four developed the facial palsy after a delay of two to eight days, and all but two recovered.

It is presumed that 'delayed facial palsy' occurs as a result of swelling or haemorrhage in or around the nerve, and those most likely to develop it have had bleeding from the ear in association with a fractured petrous temporal bone. Despite the good prognosis for delayed facial palsy, Briggs and Potter (1971) have suggested that patients with bleeding from the ears should have prophylactic ACTH. Such treatment in their hands, in a series of patients with fractured petrous temporal bones and bleeding from the ears, reduced the incidence of delayed palsy to eight per cent from the expected 20 to 40 per cent. All of their patients made a good recovery. Their experience contrasts sharply with that of Puvanendran, Vitharana and Wong (1977), who have suggested that the prognosis in delayed facial palsy is so poor as to warrant surgical decompression.

In the Newcastle series, seven patients suffered facial nerve damage; in six it was unilateral and in one bilateral. The latter patient (Case 276) suffered a severe head injury in a road accident, with resulting post-traumatic amnesia of over a week. He had extensive fractures involving the floor of the anterior cranial fossa, the middle third of the face, and the roof and margins of the orbit on both sides. He had bilateral anosmia and cerebrospinal fluid rhinorrhoea which eventually ceased spontaneously. The bilateral facial weakness was noted from the time of admission to hospital, but by six months it had completely resolved.

Of the six patients in our series with unilateral facial palsies, two developed them immediately after injury; in both instances the lesion was partial and they recovered completely. The remaining four patients developed delayed palsies; all had had bleeding from the ear on the appropriate side. One was left with a severe paresis, but the remaining three recovered almost completely even though they had suffered severe residual conductive hearing loss on the side of the facial palsy. One also had severe post-traumatic vertigo.

Out of a total of 30 patients in our study recorded to have bleeding from the ear the incidence of 'delayed facial palsy' was 13 per cent.

Eighth Cranial Nerve Injuries

In Chapter Ten we shall be dealing in detail with the problem of post-traumatic dizziness. Here we are concerned solely with hearing impairment, which is a common complication of head injury. We have already noted the frequency of aural bleeding, which so often implies otological damage. The frequency of hearing impairment after head injury has been assessed at six to eight per cent (Russell, 1960; Mealey, 1968). The majority of patients have had fractures of the petrous temporal bone although these can often be hard to detect on routine skull x-rays (Potter, 1972, 1973). Two types of temporal bone fracture are recognized (Schuknecht, 1969): the transverse variety, which goes through the anterior part of the vestibule and the basal turn of the cochlea and causes total hearing loss, and the longitudinal, which does not usually involve the labyrinthine capsule. In the latter any inner ear changes are probably attributable to concussion, and hearing loss is likely to be partial.

Partial and total hearing loss after injury occur with about equal frequency. In cases of partial deafness due to cochlear or eighth nerve damage, tinnitus may be very troublesome and for some patients more disabling than the impairment of hearing (Proctor, Gurdjian and Webster, 1956). Unfortunately nothing can be done for nerve deafness resulting from a head injury, and recovery is exceptional.

There is an extensive literature on the subject of middle ear trauma and conductive deafness resulting from head injury in the specialized otological journals. Chalat (1971) has described the various pathological processes and mechanisms involved. The most common lesion is a dysarticulation of the long process of the incus from the head of the stapes (Jackson and Magi, 1966; Hough and Stuart, 1968). It is important to recognize this lesion because it may be repaired surgically and Armstrong (1972) makes a plea for early exploration of all traumatic perforations of the ear-drum where there is associated conductive hearing loss. Frew (1970) suggests that late development of conductive deafness is a result of scar tissue involving the ossicles. Here too surgical exploration may be worthwhile.

Sixteen patients in the Newcastle series had hearing loss due to their head injuries. Four had significant nerve deafness (Table 7.7) and in one (Case 276) it was bilateral. Another patient (Case 152) had a severe crush injury with extensive skull fractures, but only a short period of post-traumatic amnesia. In addition to complete right-sided deafness which did not recover he had profound vertigo, which was attributed to associated damage to the labyrinth.

Table 7.7.   Nerve deafness (Newcastle series).

Case No.	Bleeding ear	Post-traumatic amnesia	Fracture	Side	Other features	Degree
152	—	30 minutes (crush injury)	'Every bone of skull'	R	Dizziness	Complete
179	—	5 minutes	—	L	—	Partial
228	R	Nil (crush injury)	R. parietal	R	R. VII nerve palsy	Partial
276	R	1 week	Extensive basal and facial	Bilateral	Anosmia Bilateral VII nerve palsy	Partial

Twelve patients had conductive hearing loss and all had bled from the affected ear (Table 7.8). Their head injuries varied in severity, as measured by the duration of post-traumatic amnesia. Three of them developed a delayed facial palsy and three had post-traumatic positional vertigo. In eight patients the hearing loss was partial, and most improved spontaneously. Two were thought initially to have complete conductive loss; both showed spontaneous improvement. One patient had complete hearing loss which did not improve and one had complete hearing loss that improved after surgery (Case 397). At exploratory tympanotomy, complete dislocation of the incostapedial joint was found.

Lower Cranial Nerve (9th, 10th, 11th and 12th) Injuries

The lower cranial nerves are well protected and they are damaged only in severe injuries with extensive basal skull fractures or in penetrating wounds. Collet (1915) was the first to describe injury to these nerves and his name is still associated with the syndrome of combined 9th, 10th, 11th and 12th nerve lesions. His original case had suffered a shrapnel wound at the base of the skull. Other isolated cases have been described; the topic is well reviewed by Fishbone (1976).

The foregoing paragraphs have been concerned with complications of head injury which are immediately apparent, or at least develop within hours or days of injury. We shall now consider a complication that may not appear for months or years and may well become worse with the passage of time, namely epilepsy.

Table 7.8. Conductive hearing loss (Newcastle series).

Case No.	Bleeding ear	Post-traumatic amnesia	Fracture	Side	Other signs	Degree
118	L	Not known	—	L	Positional nystagmus and vertigo. Delayed VII nerve palsy	Partial
122	L	6 days	L. basal	L	—	Partial
189	R	Nil (crush injury)	Basal	R	—	Improved Partial
196	L	20 minutes	—	L	—	Improved Complete
199	L	10 minutes	L. temporal	L	Delayed VII nerve palsy	Improved Partial
214	R	24 hours	—	R	Delayed VII nerve palsy	Improved Complete
225	L	24 hours	L. temporal	L	—	Permanent Partial
325	L	Not known	—	L	—	Permanent Partial
338	R	Nil	—	R	—	Partial
388	L	Nil	—	L	Positional nystagmus and vertigo	Complete Improved
397	R	2 hours	—	R	Positional nystagmus and vertigo	Complete Improved following surgery
409	L	Not known	—	L	—	Partial

POST-TRAUMATIC EPILEPSY

Why 'scars of the brain' should produce the abnormal neuronal excitability which is manifest as an epileptic seizure is uncertain. But the association between head injury and epilepsy has been recognized for many years, so too has the fact that the worse the injury the higher the risk of epilepsy. Much has been written on the subject of post-traumatic epilepsy; the interested reader is referred to the Symposium on Post-Traumatic Epilepsy published in *Epilepsia* (1970) to the relevant chapter in the *Late Effects of Head Injury* by Walker, Caveness and Critchley (1969) and to the excellent book by Jennett (1975).

The reported incidence of post-traumatic epilepsy varies, but this largely reflects the differences in case selection. In closed head injuries occurring in civilian life the incidence is generally accepted as 5 per cent (Jennett, 1975). In penetrating injuries of the type incurred in warfare it has been put as high as 45 per cent (Russell and Whitty, 1952; Russell and Davies-Jones, 1969). The crucial factor in penetrating injuries seems to be the depth of penetration. Caveness (1966) has suggested that the incidence of epilepsy is only 20 per cent where the dura is intact, as compared with 40 per cent in patients with dural penetration. Another factor which appears to influence the likelihood of epilepsy after penetrating wounds is the site of injury (Russell and Whitty, 1952; Caveness, 1966; Walker and Erculei, 1969; Nuutilo and Huusko, 1972; Weiss and Caveness, 1972). Thus parietal injuries appear to be followed by epilepsy more frequently than are injuries at other sites. Prolonged unconsciousness after a penetrating head injury is another factor which seems to increase the chances of subsequent epilepsy.

Post-traumatic seizures are conveniently divided into three categories based on the time of onset after injury. A seizure occurring within minutes or seconds of an injury is classified as 'immediate' and about one per cent of patients having a closed head injury will suffer this complication. A seizure in the first week after a head injury is now generally regarded as a manifestation of 'early epilepsy' and it occurs in five per cent of closed head injuries (Jennett, 1974). The third category — 'late epilepsy' — is also encountered in five per cent of closed head injuries. In neurological practice epilepsy generally implies repeated seizures, but in the context of head injuries even a single seizure may prompt the diagnosis of post-traumatic epilepsy. Early seizures are more commonly focal than late seizures, though temporal lobe attacks (complex partial seizures) in the first week after injury are uncommon.

One of the most difficult aspects of post-traumatic epilepsy — and one on which the physician is often asked to opine for medico-legal purposes — is the prediction of the likelihood of its development in an individual case. In closed head injury a number of factors have been identified that seem to be of particular influence in the possible development of post-traumatic epilepsy. One such factor is the occurrence of 'early epilepsy', which is a strong pointer to the likelihood of the development of 'late epilepsy' (Jennett, 1974, 1975). Jennett's figures provide convincing evidence of an increased incidence of late seizures in those who have had them in the first week after injury. Patients with no early seizures, no intracranial haematoma and no depressed fracture have an incidence of 'late epilepsy' of only one per cent, whereas the incidence in those patients with early seizures and depressed fractures is no less than 40 per cent.

Other factors that correlate with 'late epilepsy' are prolonged post-traumatic amnesia of greater than 12 hours, evidence of a neurological deficit and evidence of subarachnoid or other intracranial bleeding (Jennett, 1975). Jennett, Teather and Bennie (1973) have produced evidence to suggest that it is possible to predict risks of late epilepsy as early as one week after injury, using actuarial techniques. It is of interest that the electroencephalogram is of little value in predicting whether or not epilepsy will develop (Jennett, 1975). The majority of patients who are going to develop post-traumatic epilepsy will have their first seizure within five years of the injury, although occasional cases have been documented with a time lapse of greater than five years. Usually these have been patients with penetrating injuries. Whilst it is difficult to fix a cut-off point beyond which patients are safe from risks of post-traumatic epilepsy it is generally accepted that the chance of developing it are small after an interval of five years.

Certain differences may be noted when comparing post-traumatic epilepsy in children and in adults. Early fits are more common in children and tend to occur with milder injuries than might be expected to produce seizures in adults, particularly when the child is under the age of five (Jennett, 1974). Furthermore, children under 16 years are less liable to develop late epilepsy after depressed fractures than are adults (Jennett, 1975). Finally, it has been suggested that late epilepsy may develop after a longer interval in children than in adults (Mealey, 1968).

The clinical features of post-traumatic epilepsy do not differ from epilepsy due to other causes and the implications for the patient are also similar. The most serious are socioeconomic consequences, particularly in relation to occupation. Life expectancy is said to be reduced in patients who have suffered head injury, and more so in those with post-traumatic epilepsy (Walker and Erculei, 1969; Walker et al, 1971).

Interest has been focused on the routine prophylactic use of anticonvulsants after head injury to reduce the incidence of post-traumatic epilepsy, but no definite evidence of benefit has emerged (Kristiansen, Henriksen and Ringkjob, 1969; Rish and Caveness, 1973; Jennett, 1974). Anticonvulsant therapy will control attacks in most patients with post-traumatic epilepsy, but occasionally surgical treatment has been recommended (Rassmussen, 1969). There is no evidence that post-traumatic epilepsy itself is more difficult to control than other forms of symptomatic epilepsy.

In most instances the diagnosis of post-traumatic epilepsy is straightforward but sometimes there are difficulties, particularly when there are medico-legal implications. Occasionally patients will conceal the fact that fits antedated their head injury and claim that their epilepsy is a consequence of it. Or they may claim that epilepsy has been exacerbated by their injury. Frank simulation of epilepsy has been reported (Miller and Cartlidge, 1972) and, of course, other types of blackouts may be difficult to distinguish from true epilepsy (Osler and Fusillo, 1965).

As the majority of patients in the Newcastle series suffered minor head injuries, the incidence of epilepsy was low. It is of interest that nine of our patients had suffered epileptic seizures prior to their head injury and in four of these cases the head injury was directly attributable to a seizure. Two patients in the series suffered an immediate seizure and by the two-year follow-up neither had developed late epilepsy. Two others developed early epilepsy and both of these suffered further seizures within six months. Thus by Jennett's criteria there were four patients with early epilepsy, two of whom went on to develop late epilepsy.

Five patients who had had no early seizures went on to develop late epilepsy, one within the first year of injury and the other four between one and two years after injury. Thus at the end of the two-year follow-up we had a total of seven patients with post-traumatic epilepsy. All had post-traumatic amnesia of greater than 12 hours, two had had evidence of traumatic subarachnoid haemorrhage, two had had depressed skull fractures and one a subdural haematoma. Though numbers are small they tend to tally with the trends we have described.

It is perhaps worth noting here that while in coma five of our patients had intermittent focal seizures that were thought clinically not to be tonic fits. All five of these patients died and at autopsy two were shown to have extensive cortical lacerations. We believe that focal fits during head injury coma constitute a bad prognostic sign.

MISCELLANEOUS DISORDERS

In this chapter we have tried to cover the main neurological deficits and disorders that result from head injury. The list is not complete. There are a number of rarities in the literature, but sometimes in isolated cases it is difficult to decide if the condition was definitely attributable to the injury or was simply unmasked by it. Nevertheless there are a few miscellaneous disorders that should be mentioned.

Cerebral Oedema

The development of cerebral oedema in the early stages after a severe head injury is a well-recognized phenomenon both clinically and pathologically. It may subside quite quickly, but a more prolonged cerebral swelling which is indistinguishable from benign intracranial hypertension has been described as an after-effect (Beller, 1964). Patients with this syndrome are sometimes found to have had a traumatic venous sinus thrombosis.

Tumours and Cysts

It is generally believed that head injury may predispose to the development of a brain tumour, and the subject has been well reviewed by Walsh and Gye (1976). Chronic arachnoid cysts can certainly result from head injury which may either have been minor or have occurred in childhood many years previously (Tiberin and Gruszkiewicz, 1961).

Communicating Hydrocephalus

When this occurs, it is usually in patients whose head injury has been complicated by a traumatic subarachnoid haemorrhage. There is interference with absorption of cerebrospinal fluid by arachnoid villi. Patients may present at a late stage with the clinical picture of 'normal pressure hydrocephalus'. Other patients may be encountered who have hydrocephalus *ex vacuo*. These are patients who have suffered severe brain injuries with gross loss of neurones.

Effects of Skull Damage

Complications may arise as a result of damage to the skull and other structures, without significant brain damage. In the Newcastle series, there were 88 surviving patients in whom skull fractures were demonstrated. Fractures are often of little significance and they do not of themselves call for particular treatment unless they are depressed. Extradural haematomas can often be regarded as complications of skull fracture, and cerebrospinal fluid rhinorrhoea falls into the same category. It may lead to intracranial infection and sometimes to pneumocephalus.

One syndrome of childhood deserves special mention. It is the so-called 'growing fracture of the skull' (Kingsley, Till and Hoare, 1978). In this condition, serial x-rays of the head show gradual enlargement of the defect in the skull bone.

Spinal Injuries

Head injuries are not infrequently associated with spinal injuries. Two per cent of patients in the Newcastle series had spinal injuries. There is also the danger here that pre-existing but undetected myelopathy due to cervical spondylosis may produce signs that are attributed to brain injury. Four patients in our own series were found to have signs that we ascribed to pre-existing cervical spondylosis.

Damage to Blood Vessels

We have already referred to venous sinus thrombosis and the syndrome of benign intracranial hypertension. Carotico-cavernous fistula is a rare complication of head injury and there are a number of reports of aneurysms which, rightly or wrongly, have been attributed to head injury. Direct injuries to blood vessels can undoubtedly cause thrombosis and major cerebral infarction can result from direct trauma to the neck causing internal carotid artery thrombosis.

Maxillo-facial Injuries

Damage to the soft tissues of the face and to the facial bones is a common accompaniment of head injury. In the Newcastle series, 99 patients had some form of facial injury and it was a major complication in 31, of whom nine had primary orbital injuries. The subject of facial injuries is reviewed by de Jong (1975).

REFERENCES

Armstrong, B. W. (1972) Traumatic perforations of the tympanic membrane: observe or repair? *The Laryngoscope,* **82,** 1822-1830.

Arseni, C., Constantinovici, A., Iliescu, D., Dobrotă, I. & Gagea, A. (1970) Considerations on post traumatic aphasia in peace time. *Psychiatria Neurologia Neurochirugia,* **73,** 105-112.

Arne, L. (1975) Post traumatic cerebellar signs and symptoms. In *Handbook of Clinical Neurology* (Ed.) Vinken, P. J. & Bruyn, G. W. Volume **23,** pp. 459-464. Amsterdam, Oxford: North Holland Publishing. New York: American Elsevier Publishing.

Baddeley, A. D. & Patterson, K. (1971) The Relation between long term and short term memory. *British Medical Bulletin,* **27,** 237-242.

Beller, A. J. (1964) Benign post traumatic intracranial hypertension. *Journal of Neurology, Neurosurgery and Psychiatry,* **27,** 149-152.

Bodian, M. (1964) Transient loss of vision following head trauma. *New York State Journal of Medicine,* **64,** 916-920.

Bricolo, A. (1976) Prolonged post traumatic coma. In *Handbook of Clinical Neurology* (Ed.) Vinken, P. J. & Bruyn, G. W. Volume **24,** pp. 699-756. Amsterdam, Oxford: North Holland Publishing. New York: American Elsevier Publishing.

Briggs, M. & Potter, J. M. (1971) Prevention of delayed traumatic facial palsy. *British Medical Journal,* **iii,** 458-459.

Brock, S. (1960) *Injuries of the Brain and Spinal Cord and their Coverings.* London: Cassell.

Brooks, D. N. (1976) Wechsler-Memory scale performance and its relationship to brain injury after severe closed head injury. *Journal of Neurology, Neurosurgery and Psychiatry,* **39,** 593-601.

Burger, L. J., Kalvin, N. H. & Lawton Smith, J. (1970) Acquired lesions of the fourth cranial nerve. *Brain,* **93,** 567-574.

Caplan, L. R. & Zervas, N. T. (1977) Survival with permanent mid brain dysfunction after surgical treatment of traumatic sub dural haematoma: the clinical picture of a Duret haemorrhage. *Annals of of Neurology,* **1,** 587-589.

Caveness, W. F. (1966) Post traumatic sequelae. In *Head Injury* (Ed.) Caveness, W. F. & Walker, A. E. pp. 209-219. Philadelphia and Toronto: J. B. Lippincott.

Chalat, N. I. (1971) Middle ear effect of head trauma. *The Laryngoscope,* **81,** 1286-1303.

Chapman, L. I., Urist, M. J., Folk, E. R. & Miller, M. T. (1970) Acquired bilateral superior oblique muscle palsy. *Archives of Ophthalmology,* **84,** 137-142.

Collet, S. (1915) Sur un nouveau syndrome paralytique pharyngolarynge par blessure de guerre. *Lyon Medical,* **124,** 121-129.

Crompton, M. R., Teare, R. D. & Bowen, D. A. L. (1966) Prolonged coma after head injury. *Lancet,* **ii,** 938-940.

Crompton, M. R. (1970) Visual lesions in closed head injury. *Brain,* **93,** 785-792.

Crompton, M. R. (1971) Brain stem lesions due to closed head injury. *Lancet,* **i,** 669-673.

Cullen, J. F. (1964) Occlusion of the central retinal artery following a closed head injury. *American Journal of Ophthalmology,* **57,** 670-672.

de Jong, B. D. (1975) Craniofacial Injuries. *Handbook of Clinical Neurology* (Ed.) Vinken, P. J. & Bruyn, G. W. Amsterdam, Oxford: North Holland Publishing. New York: American Elsevier Publishing.

Fahy, T. J., Irving, M. H. & Millac, P. (1967) Severe head injuries. *Lancet,* **ii,** 475-479.

Feiring, E. H. (1974) *'Brocks' Injuries of the Brain and Spinal Cord* Fifth Edition. New York: Springer Publishing.

Fisher, A. (1965) Arachnoiditis in the chiasmatic cistern following head injury with reference to the pneumographic diagnosis. *Proceedings of the Eighth International Congress of Neurology,* 341-344.

Fisher, C. M. (1966) Concussion amnesia. *Neurology,* **16,** 826-830.

Fishbone, H. (1976) Irreversible injury of the last four cranial nerves. In *Handbook of Clinical Neurology* (Ed.) Vinken, P. J. & Bruyn, G. W. Volume **24.** pp. 179-181. Amsterdam, Oxford: North Holland Publishing. New York: American Elsevier Publishing.

Frew, I. J. C. (1970) Delayed conductive deafness. *Journal of Laryngology and Otology,* **84,** 939-941.

Gjerris, F. (1976) Traumatic lesions of the visual pathways. In *Handbook of Clinical Neurology* (Ed.) Vinken, P. J. & Bruyn, G. W. Volume **24.** pp. 27-58. Amsterdam, Oxford: North Holland Publishing. New York: American Elsevier Publishing.

Glaser, M. A. & Shafer, F. P. (1932) Skull and brain traumas: their sequelae. *Journal of the American Medical Association,* **98,** 271-276.

Goland, P. P. (1937) Olfactometry in cases of acute head injury. *Archives of Surgery,* **35,** 1173-1182.

Griffith, J. F. & Dodge, P. R. (1968) Transient blindness following head injury in children. *New England Journal of Medicine,* **278,** 648-651.

Hagan, P. J. (1967) Post traumatic anosmia. *Archives of Otolaryngology,* **85,** 107-111.

Hart, C. T. (1969) Disturbances of fusion following head injury. *Proceedings of the Royal Society of Medicine,* **62,** 704-706.

Hermann, K. (1965) Post traumatic dysarthria. In *The Proceedings of the Eighth International Congress of Neurology* pp. 135-138. Verlag der Wiener Medizinischen Akademie.

Heilman, K. M., Safran, A. & Geschwind, N. (1971) Closed head trauma and aphasia. *Journal of Neurology, Neurosurgery and Psychiatry,* **34,** 265-269.

Hough, J. V. D. & Stuart, W. D. (1968) Middle ear injuries in skull trauma. *Laryngoscope,* **78,** 899-936.

Hughes, B. (1954) *The Visual Fields.* Oxford: Blackwell.

Hughes, B. (1962) Indirect injury of the optic nerve and chiasma. *Bulletin of the Johns Hopkins Hospital,* **111,** 98-126.

Humphrey, M. E. & Zangwill, O. L. (1951) Cessation of dreaming after brain injury. *Journal of Neurology, Neurosurgery and Psychiatry,* **14,** 322-325.

Jackson, J. H. (1864) Illustrations of diseases of the nervous system. *London Hospital Reports,* **1,** 337-341.

Jackson, F. E. & Magi, M. (1966) Traumatic dislocation of the incus associated with basilar skull fracture. *Journal of Neurosurgery,* **24,** 570-572.

Jellinger, K. & Seitelberger, F. (1970) Protracted post traumatic encephalopathy; pathology, pathogenesis and clinical implications. *Journal of the Neurological Sciences,* **10,** 51-94.

Jennett, B. & Plum, F. (1972) Persistent vegetative state after brain damage. *Lancet,* **i,** 734-737.

Jennett, W. B. (1974) Early traumatic epilepsy. *Archives of Neurology,* **30,** 394-398.

Jennett, W. B. (1975) *Epilepsy after Non Missile Head Injuries.* Second Edition. London: William Heinemann Medical Books.

Jennett, W. B. (1976) Prognosis after head injury. In *Handbook of Clinical Neurology* (Ed.) Uinken, P. J. & Bruyn, G. W. Volume 24, pp. 669-682. Amsterdam, Oxford: North Holland Publishing. New York: American Elsevier Publishing.

Jennett, W. B., Teather, D. & Bennie, S. (1973) Epilepsy after head injury. *Lancet,* **ii,** 652-653.

Jooma, O. V. (1972) The problem of brain stem injury with special reference to serial EEG studies, long term rehabilitation and results. *Scandinavian Journal of Rehabilitation Medicine,* **4,** 100-105.

Keane, J. R. (1975) Ocular skew deviation. *Archives of Neurology,* **32,** 185-190.

Kingsley, D., Till, K. & Hoare, R. (1978) Growing fractures of the skull. *Journal of Neurology, Neurosurgery and Psychiatry,* **41,** 312-318.

Kremer, M., Russell, W. R. & Smyth, G. E. (1947) A mid brain syndrome following head injury. *Journal of Neurology, Neurosurgery and Psychiatry,* **10,** 49-60.

Kristiansen, K., Henriksen, G. F. & Ringkjob, R. (1969) Traumatic epilepsy: prophylaxis. In *The Late Effects of Head Injury* (Ed.) Walker, A. E., Caveness, W. F. & Critchley, M. pp. 261-276. Springfield, Illinois: C. C. Thomas.

Leigh, A. D. (1943) Defects of smell after head injury. *Lancet,* **i,** 38-40.

Levin, H. S., Grossman, R. G. & Kelly, P. J. (1976) Aphasic disorder in patients with closed head injury. *Journal of Neurology, Neurosurgery and Psychiatry,* **39,** 1062-1070.

Mealey, J. (1968) *Paediatric Head Injuries.* Springfield, Illinois: C. C. Thomas.

Merritt, H. H. (1943) Head Injury. Review of the literature. *War Medicine,* **4,** 61-82, 187-215.

Miller, H. & Stern, G. (1965) The long term prognosis of severe head injury. *Lancet,* **i,** 225-229.

Miller, H. & Cartlidge, N. E. F. (1972) Simulation and malingering after injuries to the brain and spinal cord. *Lancet,* **i,** 580-585.

Mitchell, D. E. & Adams, J. H. (1973) Primary focal impact damage to the brain stem in blunt head injuries. Does it exist? *Lancet,* **ii,** 215-218.

Newcombe, F., Oldfield, R. C., Ratcliff, G. G. & Wingfield, A. (1971) Recognition and naming of object-drawings by men with focal brain wounds. *Journal of Neurology, Neurosurgery and Psychiatry,* **34,** 329-340.

Nuutilo, A. & Huusko, S. (1972) Epilepsy among brain injured veterans; twenty six to thirty one years following the injury. *Scandinavian Journal of Rehabilitation Medicine,* **4,** 81-84.

Osler, L. D. & Fusillo, M. G. (1965) A peculiar type of post concussive blackout. *Journal of Neurology, Neurosurgery and Psychiatry,* **28,** 344-349.

Potter, G. D. (1973) Trauma of the ear. *Otolaryngologic Clinics of North America*, **6**, 401-412.

Potter, G. D. (1972) Temporal bone fractures — problems in radiologic diagnosis. *Laryngoscope*, **82**, 408-413.

Proctor, B., Gurdjian, E. S. & Webster, J. E. (1956) The ear in head trauma. *Laryngoscope*, **66**, 16-61.

Puvanendran, K., Vitharana, M. & Wong, P. K. (1977) Delayed facial palsy after head injury. *Journal of Neurology, Neurosurgery and Psychiatry*, **40**, 342-350.

Rassmussen, T. (1969) Surgical Therapy of post traumatic epilepsy. In *The Late Effects of Head Injury* (Ed.) Walker, A. E., Caveness, W. F. & Critchley, M. pp. 277-305. Springfield, Illinois: C. C. Thomas.

Rish, B. L. & Caveness, W. F. (1973) Relation of prophylactic medication to the occurrence of early seizures following cranio cerebral trauma. *Journal of Neurosurgery*, **38**, 155-158.

Roberts, M. & Owens, G. (1972) Delayed traumatic bilateral abducens paralysis without skull fracture or brain injury. *Journal of Trauma*, **12**, 254-257.

Rowbotham, G. S. (1964) *Acute Injuries of the Head*. Fourth edition. Edinburgh and London: E. & S. Livingstone.

Russell, W. R. (1932) Cerebral involvement in head injury. *Brain*, **55**, 549-563.

Russell, W. R. (1935) Amnesia following head injuries. *Lancet*, **ii**, 762-763.

Russell, W. R. (1960) Injury to cranial nerves and optic chiasm. In *Injuries of the Brain and Spinal Cord and their Coverings* (Ed.) Brock, S. London: Cassell.

Russell, W. R. (1971) *The Traumatic Amnesias*. Oxford: University Press.

Russell, W. R. & Davies-Jones, G. A. B. (1969) Epilepsy following the brain wounds of World War II. In *The Late Effects of Head Injury*. (Ed.) Walker, A. E., Caveness, W. F. & Critchley, M. pp. 189-192. Springfield, Illinois: C. C. Thomas.

Russell, W. R. & Espir, M. L. E. (1961) *Traumatic Aphasia*. London: Oxford University Press.

Russell, W. R. & Nathan, P. W. (1946) Traumatic amnesia. *Brain*, **69**, 280-300.

Russell, W. R. & Smith, A. (1961) Post traumatic amnesia in closed head injury. *Archives of Neurology*, **5**, **426-429**.

Russell, W. R. & Whitty, C. W. M. (1952) Studies in traumatic epilepsy; 1. factors influencing the incidence of epilepsy after brain wounds. *Journal of Neurology, Neurosurgery and Psychiatry*, **15**, 93-98.

Sabin, T. D. & Poche, J. A. (1969) Pure tortional nystagmus as a consequence of head trauma. *Journal of Neurology, Neurosurgery and Psychiatry*, **32**, 265-267.

Schechter, P. J. & Henkin, R. I. (1974) Abnormalities of taste and smell after head trauma. *Journal of Neurology, Neurosurgery and Psychiatry*, **37**, 802-810.

Schneider, R. A. (1972) Anosmia; verification and aetiologies. *Annals of Otology, Rhinology and Laryngology*, **81**, 272-277.

Schuknecht, H. F. (1969) Mechanism of inner ear injury from blows to the head. *Annals of Otology*, **78**, 253-262.

Strauss, I. & Savitsky, N. (1934) Head injury; neurologic and psychiatric aspects. *Archives of Neurology and Psychiatry*, **31**, 893-954.

Strich, S. J. (1969) The pathology of brain damage due to blunt head injuries. In *The Late Effects of Head Injury* (Ed.) Walker, A. E., Caveness, W. F. & Critchley, M. pp. 501-528. Springfield, Illinois: C. C. Thomas.

Sumner, D. (1964) Post traumatic anosmia. *Brain*, **7**, 107-120.

Sumner, D. (1976) Disturbance of the senses of smell and taste after head injuries. In *Handbook of Clinical Neurology* (Ed.) Vinken, P. J. & Bruyn, G. W. Volume **24**, pp. 1-26. Amsterdam, Oxford: North Holland Publishing. New York: American Elsevier Publishing.

Symonds, C. P. (1960) Concussion and contusion of the brain and their sequelae. In *Injuries of the Brain and Spinal Cord and their Coverings*. (Ed.) Brock, S. pp. 69-117. London: Cassell.

Symposium on Post Traumatic Epilepsy (1970) *Epilepsia*, **11**, 5-94.

Thomsen, I. V. (1975) Evaluation and outcome of aphasia in patients with severe closed head trauma. *Journal of Neurology, Neurosurgery and Psychiatry*, **38**, 713-718.

Tiberin, P. & Gruszkiewicz, J. (1961) Chronic arachnoidal cysts of the middle cranial fossa and their relation to trauma. *Journal of Neurology, Neurosurgery and Psychiatry*, **24**, 86-91.

Traquair, H. M., Dott, N. M. & Russell, W. R. (1935) Traumatic lesions of the optic chiasma. *Brain*, **58**, 398-411.

Turner, J. W. A. (1943) Indirect injuries of the optic nerve. *Brain*, **66**, 140-151.

Turner, J. W. A. (1944) Facial palsy in closed head injuries. *Lancet*, **i**, 756-757.

Walker, A. E. and Erculei, F. (1969) *Head injured men; fifteen years later*. Springfield, Illinois: C. C. Thomas.

Walker, A. E., Leuchs, H. K., Lechpape-Gruter, H., Caveness, W. F. & Kretschman, C. (1971) Life expectancy of head injured men with and without epilepsy. **24**, 95-100.

Wallace, A. (1969) Speech disorders following head injury. *Injury*, **1**, 140-143.

Walsh, J. and Gye, R. (1976) Traumatic meningioma. In *Handbook of Clinical Neurology.* (Ed.) Vinken, P. J. & Bruyn, G. W. Volume **24**, pp. 441-444. Amsterdam, Oxford: North Holland Publishing. New York: American Elsevier Publishing.

Wasterlain, C. G. (1971) Are there two types of post traumatic retrograde amnesia? *European Neurology,* **5**, 225-228.

Weiss, G. H. & Caveness, W. F. (1972) Prognostic factors in the persistence of post traumatic epilepsy. *Journal of Neurosurgery,* **37**, 164-169.

Weisz, G. M., Hemli, L. & Kraus, J. J. (1975) Transient blindness following minor head injuries. *Injury,* **6**, 348-350.

Williams, M. & Zangwill, O. L. (1952) Memory defects after head injury. *Journal of Neurology, Neurosurgery and Psychiatry,* **15**, 54-58.

Wolpaw, J. R. (1971) The aetiology of retrograde amnesia. *Lancet,* **ii**, 356-357.

Wyllie, A. M., McLeod, D. & Cullen, J. F. (1972) Traumatic ischaemic optic neuropathy. *British Journal of Ophthalmology,* **56**, 851-853.

Yarnell, P. R. & Lynch, S. (1970) Retrograde memory immediately after concussion. *Lancet,* **i**, 863-864.

Yin, R. K. (1970) Face recognition by brain injured patients: a dissociable ability? *Neuropsychologia,* **8**, 395-402.

CHAPTER EIGHT

The Psychiatric Sequelae of Head Injury

A coherent review of the literature on the psychiatric and psychological aspects of head injury is hindered by variation and inconsistency in the definitions and classifications used by writers on the subject, but these factors alone cannot be held responsible for all the differing interpretations that emerge. As in many other fields of clinical research, at least some of the discrepancies result from variations in the source and characteristics of the populations studied. Several disciplines are involved. The psychiatrist and the neurosurgeon, for instance, are unlikely to collect, for special study, groups of patients without some inherent sampling differences: nor will it be surprising if they sometimes reach different conclusions from the same observations, bearing in mind the lack of uniformity of their training and experience. But there is an additional factor which colours and indeed enlivens the literature on the subject. It would be unfair to call it prejudice but some of the best writing does carry a mark of conviction that transcends the supporting evidence.

Differences in terminology, although confusing, are not of paramount importance. There is only a limited number of clinical phenomena falling within the general category under consideration and, whatever the definition or classification adopted by an individual author, it is usually possible to identify the particular class of defect or abnormality to which he is referring. Table 8.1 lists the various types of psychiatric or psychological sequelae that may be encountered after head injury, without attempting to organize them into a logical or structured classification. It may seem strange, particularly to the neurologist, that dementia is included under the heading of 'post-traumatic psychoses'. Most neurologists make a clear distinction between dementia — an organic disorder of the brain due to injury or disease causing disintegration of memory and intellect, and psychosis — allegedly a disorder of the mind. But in most of the psychiatric literature such a precise distinction is not maintained; dementia is usually classified as an organic psychosis, in contrast to those other disorders with no demonstrable structural or biochemical abnormality, which are classified as functional.

Some of the items in Table 8.1 are encountered only infrequently but all are relatively easy to identify. What is not easy to determine, and indeed constitutes the main subject of controversy, is the precise mechanism whereby the symptom or symptoms may be produced by the head injury and in particular whether or not they are mediated by some structural alteration, however subtle.

There are many references in the literature to the interplay of psychological and organic factors that predispose to the development of late symptoms following head injury. The psychological determinants are well established largely on the basis of studies carried out during and after the Second World War. Lishman (1968) has listed many of them, along with the authors attesting them. They include the

Table 8.1.   Psychological and psychiatric syndromes after head injury.

Syndrome
Amnesia
Retrograde
Post-traumatic
Postconcussional syndrome
Post-traumatic neurosis
Post-traumatic hysteria
Post-traumatic psychosis
Personality/behavioural change
Confusion/delirium
Dementia
Schizophrenia
Depression
Mania

This table should be read in conjunction with the text on page 81.

individual's mental constitution (Symonds and Russell, 1943; Dencker, 1958, 1960), factors in the premorbid personality (Kozol, 1945, 1946), conflicts little related to the injury (Ruesch and Bowman, 1945), the emotional reaction to the injury itself (Denny-Brown, 1945; Guttmann, 1946), the psychological response to intellectual impairment (Goldstein, 1952), environmental difficulties (Adler, 1945; Kozol, 1945, 1946) and factors of compensation or litigation (Kozol, 1945, 1946; Miller, 1961).

This is a formidable list of variables; any (or indeed all) of them may be relevant to the aftermath of a head injury. They are certainly liable to cloud the issue when attempts are made to identify the physical determinants of psychiatric sequelae. As Lishman puts it, 'brain damage has to compete with all of them for a place in the aetiological hierarchy'. The difficulty has always been the lack of precise methods of measuring the extent of physical brain damage during life, and the obvious lack of pathological data in all but the most severe cases. An important step forward was the recognition by Russell (1968) that the severity of injury in organic terms can be assessed with some degree of accuracy by measurement of the length of post-traumatic amnesia. This correlation, together with other aspects of organic brain damage, was discussed in Chapters Six and Seven.

Whilst both psychological and physical determinants of the sequelae of head injury have been studied extensively and with some degree of success, the central dilemma remains: what is the relative role of each in the development of mental symptoms in an individual who has suffered head injury? The point will be returned to when individual psychiatric syndromes are discussed later in the chapter.

INCIDENCE OF PSYCHIATRIC SEQUELAE

The quoted incidence of psychiatric or psychological symptoms after head injury varies considerably, depending on the methods of selection of the cases studied. Ota (1965, 1969) studied 1168 adult patients after head injury and found 52 who were psychotic, 80 who had shown personality change and 250 who were suffering from some sort of neurosis. In this breakdown, 'psychosis' is used in the sense that Bowman, Blau and Reich (1974) used it — to embrace all mental disorders primarily due to trauma, including intellectual loss. These authors used the term 'neurosis' to cover mental disorders either associated with, or precipitated or complicated by head trauma, but not primarily due to it. In a study of 170 patients who had suffered severe head injury, Vigouroux et al (1972) identified 59 who had psychiatric symptoms. Thirty-one patients had memory disturbances, and 19 complained of poor concentration. Thirty-eight were diagnosed as having a neurosis; six were classified as demented, and two had schizophrenia. There were six patients thought to have a manic-depressive psychosis, and 15 were regarded as suffering from personality disorders.

One of the few prospective studies of a group of unselected head injury patients was that carried out by Denny-Brown and his colleagues in Boston in the early 1940s. Two hundred cases were examined carefully by neurologists and psychiatrists, during and after the stay in hospital, and all of them were followed up by a social worker. The results of the psychiatric assessments were published in a series of articles (Adler, 1945; Kozol, 1945, 1946). Adler (1945) reported that 63 (31.5 per cent) of the 200 patients developed post-traumatic mental symptoms and 48 of them developed an anxiety neurosis.

In the following paragraphs we will discuss briefly some of the disorders listed in Table 8.1. We would again emphasize that this list does not in any way represent an ordered classification. We have yet to find one that either simplifies or illuminates the topic under consideration, so the list simply consists of a number of conditions which are well recognized, using the names by which they are familiarly known.

AMNESIA — RETROGRADE AND POST-TRAUMATIC

These have been discussed in detail in Chapter Seven.

POSTCONCUSSIONAL SYNDROME

This important and controversial subject will be discussed in detail in Chapter Eleven, but it would seem reasonable to anticipate the main conclusions that are to be drawn. A case is made for abolishing the term altogether because of the belief that its constituent parts do not necessarily have a common aetiology. The concept of a syndrome with well-defined and presumably consistent characteristics runs the risk of obscuring the possible contribution of an organic labyrinthine affection in one patient, or of a true reactive depression in another. We would like to see each symptom analysed separately, with particular attention paid to its time of onset in relation to the injury.

POST-TRAUMATIC NEUROSIS

In general terms, neurosis may be regarded as an expression of an individual's personality and his or her reactions to the outside world. A post-traumatic neurosis is likely to be governed as much by the premorbid personality of the affected individual as by the nature and degree of the injury. Both may play a part. An extensive psychoanalytical literature has built up on the subject of post-traumatic neurosis; the following observation, attributed to Freud, is quoted by Brock (1960): 'if anxiety is the reaction of the ego to danger, then it would be the obvious thing to regard the traumatic neuroses, which are so often the sequel of exposing one's life to danger, as the direct result of life or death anxiety, . . .'. Bastin (1930), Roche (1960) and Braverman and Hacker (1965) have all provided interesting reviews on the subject. Grinker and Spiegel (1945), on the basis of their studies during the Second World War, suggested that the identification of particular types of post-traumatic neurosis was of little help. They suggested that the best way to understand the neuroses was to examine them in relation to the precipitating factors (the trauma), the predisposing factors (emotional vulnerability and ego strength) and the dynamic struggle (symptoms).

Brock (1960) wrote a helpful review of the subject of post-traumatic neurosis. He suggested that neurotic symptoms are particularly common after head injury because of man's natural concern for the well-being of his head and his brain. It is easy to accept that anxieties about impairment of brain function could contribute to the development of neurotic symptoms, particularly in those who are so predisposed. The problem is perhaps compounded by public awareness of the serious consequences of brain injury. Patients often express their worries about 'blood clots on the brain' long after the possibility of any such complication is past. Brock makes the point that the greater the amount of organic brain damage, the less likely the patient is to develop neurotic symptoms. He believes that anxiety states and conversion hysteria are the most common manifestations of neurosis after injury, and that neurasthenic, hypochondriacal and depressive states are relatively rare.

The patterns of recovery from post-traumatic neurosis are variable and unpredictable. In a detailed study of 101 patients who had suffered a head injury, Kozol (1946) found that 50 per cent still had neurotic symptoms six months after injury and 15 per cent had symptoms that persisted for a year or more. He observed no close correlation between the severity of the acute injury to the brain and the severity of the psychiatric sequelae, but he did note a correlation between continuing psychosocial problems and the persistence of symptoms. The psychosocial factors that he identified included pending litigation, continuing problems with compensation, occupational stress and persisting physical disability. He claimed (1945, 1946) that the pre-injury personality of the individual had little to do with the development or persistence of post-traumatic mental symptoms.

The basic personality of an individual may obviously influence the reaction to accident or injury. Adler (1945) reported that 50 per cent of those who develop post-traumatic anxiety have abnormal personalities even before the accident. But he also, like Kozol, believes that psychosocial factors are of importance in the perpetuation of post-traumatic symptoms.

POST-TRAUMATIC HYSTERIA

The above heading is included with some misgiving. It raises the perennial, and largely unanswerable, questions about conscious and unconscious motivation and about the distinction between hysteria and frank malingering. Miller (1961), on the basis of very wide experience, adopted an uncompromising attitude and believed that in most cases the symptoms of post-traumatic neurosis were exaggerated, or deliberately simulated, for purposes of financial gain. It would, indeed, be surprising if there was not a tendency for some patients at least to make the most of their symptoms in the hope of improving the compensation prospects, but blatant malingering seems to be comparatively uncommon. It is worth reminding ourselves just how frequently, in routine practice unconnected with accidents, we encounter patients with a so-called 'functional overlay'. It seems that if a part of the body is damaged a patient may have a generally reduced expectation of the performance of that part. In ordinary practice we are not unduly surprised by this phenomenon, but when it occurs in the postinjury setting it is tempting to assume conscious exaggeration or, less charitably, base deception. These difficult questions are discussed at greater length in Chapter Eleven, which deals with the postconcussional syndrome.

All the disorders discussed so far are subsumed under the general heading of 'neuroses' by most authors. In the following paragraphs we shall be dealing with disturbances of a different order, they fall outside the range of normal human experience and are often, in the context of head injury, collected together under the general heading of 'post-traumatic psychoses'. As already indicated, we have some misgivings about this broad distinction, particularly in view of the lack of consistency in its interpretation by different authors. Nevertheless, because it is a classification which has been so widely adopted we will continue to employ it for purposes of description.

POST-TRAUMATIC PSYCHOSES

The reported incidence of post-traumatic psychosis varies considerably, depending largely on the selection of cases. Ota (1965) found an incidence of 2.7 per cent in his series of 1168 adults admitted to hospital with closed head injuries. Hillbom and Jarho (1969) studied a series of Finnish war veterans who had suffered head injury and found that 8.9 per cent of them developed a psychosis. Miller and Stern (1965), in a study of 100 head-injured patients with post-traumatic amnesia of greater than 24 hours, found ten in the psychotic category — all with dementia. Among 32 patients with severe head injury, Fahy, Irving and Millac (1967) encountered only five who were totally free of psychiatric symptoms.

As already indicated, there are many different ways of splitting up the various disorders included in the general category of psychosis. Hillbom and Jarho (1969) in their study used the classification set out in Table 8.2. Ota (1969) likewise had quite an exhaustive list of disorders within the psychotic category, but nowadays, with increasing knowledge of the relationship between psychosis and head injury, a more compact and practical classification has emerged. It recognizes four main disorder groups:

dementia/delirium   (organic psychoses)
schizophrenia
endogenous depression   } (functional psychoses)
manic states.

The relationship between each one of these and head injury is reasonably well defined. In the case of penetrating injuries, a major contribution was made by Lishman (1968). He carried out a detailed psychiatric survey of the Oxford head injury patients, whose previous study by neurologists had already yielded so much valuable information. Lishman's study was obviously based on retrospective analysis of case records, but the majority of these were of high quality. Patients were divided into three groups: those with no psychiatric disability, those with severe psychiatric disability, and a third group who were regarded as having mild psychiatric disability. He defined psychiatric disability as 'a disturbance in any area of mental life as reflected by impairment of intellectual function, disorder of affect, disorder of behaviour, somatic complaints without demonstrable physical basis, and/or formal psychiatric illness'. With the single exception of 'somatic complaints without physical cause', Lishman found a correlation between the severity of symptoms and the extent of brain damage. His series included a total of 670 patients. He used the term 'psychotic' in a restricted sense and had only five patients thus categorized. However, the series included 117 patients with intellectual impairment and 113 with affective disorders of severe degree and, in terms of the definition that we are applying, all these patients would clearly fall within the psychotic group.

Table 8.2.   Psychotic syndromes after head injury (Hillbom & Jarho, 1969).

Schizophrenic or schizophreniform
Paranoid
Epileptic
Commotio
Depressive
Korsakoff
Intoxication/delirium
Amentiform
Grave dementia

The use of the term 'commotio' in this table is obscure and is not explained in the text of the paper.

As already mentioned, Lishman's study was confined to patients who had suffered penetrating injuries and the severity of brain damage was calculated on the basis of two indices: 'depth of penetration' and 'total brain tissue destroyed'. His study clearly demonstrated a correlation between the severity of damage according to these indices and the development of psychiatric symptoms. Furthermore his figures showed that intellectual impairment and severe affective disorder were by far the most important psychiatric sequelae. The lack of correlation between the degree of brain damage and the incidence of somatic complaints without obvious organic cause tends to support the view of Miller (1961) that the postconcussional syndrome is nonorganic.

Support for Lishman's findings comes from a report by Achte, Hillbom and Aalberg (1969), from Finland. These authors drew attention to the fact that in their series the onset of psychosis was often delayed. Heiskanen and Sipponen (1970) also established the connection between severity of injury and development of psychosis (in the broadest sense of the term) in a study of 204 patients who had been unconscious for more than 24 hours after head injury. They recorded that 43 per cent of their patients were still severely disabled three years after the injury and that in the majority of cases intellectual loss was the predominant feature.

There are thus several good studies which confirm the relationship between severity of injury and degree of intellectual impairment. As regards other components within the general category of 'psychosis' that we have chosen to adopt, delirium, confusion and the amnesias have already been considered in Chapters Six and Seven. True schizophrenic psychosis resulting from head injury is obviously rare, but examples are quoted, particularly in relation to very severe injuries. Miller (1966) and Merskey and Woodforde (1972) gave instances of individuals developing schizophrenia after minor head injuries, but it seems likely that these were coincidental associations and that the head injuries had brought to light incipient mental illness. Cases of this sort do, of course, tend to raise extremely difficult medicolegal problems.

Whilst reactive depression is a common sequel of head injury, endogenous depressions are infrequently encountered, though Merskey and Woodforde (1972) have drawn attention to their occurrence. Mania is likewise a very infrequent complication. Presumably endogenous depression and mania, when they do occur, are merely precipitated by head injury in constitutionally predisposed individuals.

The majority of studies quoted and the discussion so far have been concerned with the sequelae of single injuries. However, dementia as a result of repeated head injuries is well recognized in the punch-drunk syndrome (Mawdsley & Ferguson, 1963). More recently, the occurrence of a similar syndrome in jockeys suffering repeated head injuries has been reported by Foster, Leiguarda and Tilley (1976).

NATURAL HISTORY OF PSYCHIATRIC SEQUELAE

In recent years a number of studies have added substantially to our knowledge of the natural history and the recovery prospects for psychological deficits resulting from head injury. Many of these studies have been carried out by workers in Glasgow (Brooks, 1972, 1974, 1976; Mandleberg, 1975, 1976; Mandleberg and Brooks, 1975; Bond, 1975) who have concentrated on longitudinal observations on patients with impairment of both intellectual function and memory.

A variety of psychological tests have been devised for studying the type of memory defect that may be encountered in patients with head injury. Fodor (1972) tried to evaluate a number of them but could not, on the basis of her studies, find a definite relationship between the severity of injury and the performance of patients on her memory scale. Brooks (1972), on the other hand, tested memory in a series of 27 patients with severe head injury and showed that severity was an important determinant of memory performance. This was particularly true for older patients; the association was rather less conspicuous in the young.

It was suggested by Conky (1938) and by Ruesch (1944) that recovery of memory impairment occurs within the first few months after injury. Brooks (1974, 1976) has also found that most of the recovery is completed within six months. However, he has suggested also that the functions of memory and of intelligence recover at different rates after injury (Brooks, 1976).

The Glasgow team have been particularly interested in the relationship between impairment of intellectual function and the severity of the head injury, and they have studied in detail the patterns of recovery of intellectual function. Mandleberg and Brooks (1975) have produced evidence which suggests that verbal IQ can improve progressively for up to a year after injury, whilst performance IQ can continue to improve for as long as three years. In a group of 40 patients they showed that cognitive ability eventually returned to near normal, despite the fact that the injuries had been severe (as judged by duration of post-traumatic amnesia). In a separate study in Glasgow, Mandleberg (1975) administered the Wechsler Adult Intelligence Scale (WAIS) to two matched groups of patients with severe head injuries. In one group, the patients were still in a period of extending post-traumatic amnesia, but in the second group the period of post-traumatic amnesia was fixed. As might have been expected, the WAIS was significantly lower in the patients whose post-traumatic amnesia was still extending. They were retested when their post-traumatic amnesia had stabilized and then their scores matched those of the second group. However, there were interesting differences between verbal and performance abilities: the former appeared less affected than the latter during the period of post-traumatic amnesia. Perhaps this result was not entirely unexpected, as the performance tasks of the WAIS are inherently more difficult than the verbal ones.

The duration of post-traumatic amnesia is generally regarded as a good index of severity of injury, and it has been shown to correlate with eventual cognitive level (Tooth, 1947; Russell and Smith, 1961; Lishman, 1968). Surprisingly enough, other investigators have failed to establish the relationship (Dencker and Lofving, 1958; Dencker, 1958). The experience in Glasgow, reported by Mandleberg (1976), is that three months after injury the verbal IQ level correlates with the duration of post-traumatic amnesia, but at six months the relationship can no longer be established. Performance IQ, on the other hand, was found by Mandleberg (1976) to relate to length of post-traumatic amnesia both at three months and at six months. At 12 and 30 months after injury, however, even this relationship did not hold. The conclusion reached on the basis of this study was that eventual cognitive outcome does not relate to severity of injury as measured by post-traumatic amnesia. Mandleberg's interpretation of his results is that the length of post-traumatic amnesia relates more accurately to the rate of improvement of cognitive function than to the final outcome. In this study he found no statistically significant differences between IQ scores of patients with short periods and those with long periods of post-traumatic amnesia, but it is fair to say that there was a noticeable tendency for patients with longer periods of post-traumatic amnesia to score less well. Obviously there must be a point on the head injury severity scale beyond which little recovery is likely to occur, and there is no return to normal. Bond (1975) suggests that, if the period of post-traumatic amnesia exceeds 11 weeks, there is unlikely to be complete recovery of verbal or performance IQ.

The recovery patterns for other psychological deficits after severe head injury are less well documented. Changes in personality and behaviour are not uncommon after severe injury and they may persist for a considerable time or possibly remain permanently. Patients who have previously had stable personalities may become euphoric, and may exhibit disinhibited or frankly unsocial behaviour.

In spite of the various studies referred to it must be said that, in general, the prediction of outcome of psychiatric disability after head injury is beset with difficulties. Some helpful guidelines have emerged from the extensive study reported by Lewin, Marshall and Roberts (1979), based on a consecutive series of 7000 patients with head injuries admitted to the Regional Accident Service in Oxford. The findings suggested that, in adolescence and early adult years, an injury sufficiently severe enough to produce a period of post-traumatic amnesia of from two to eight weeks is likely to result in a moderate degree of permanent mental disability. In the middle-aged and elderly, a period of post-traumatic amnesia of a month or more will usually result in severe mental disability.

NEWCASTLE SERIES

Psychiatric assessments were carried out on all patients in the Newcastle series on discharge from hospital and at the six-month, one-year and two-year follow-up. Assessments were recorded on a standard proforma and the majority were made by the same observer (N.E.F.C.). Patients were not seen routinely by a psychiatrist, but they were referred for psychiatric advice whenever this was thought to be in their best interest.

Disorders of Affect

Included in the psychiatric enquiry was an assessment of whether or not there was any disturbance of affect. Table 8.3 lists the five descriptive categories used within the general group of affective disorders and indicates the number of patients in each category on discharge and at the follow-up intervals. The two most common types of disturbance were depression and anxiety.

Table 8.3. Disorders of affect (Newcastle series).

	No. of cases			
Disorder	On discharge	After 6 months	After 1 year	After 2 years
Depression	31	60	58	56
Emotional lability	4	8	5	4
Anxiety	30	40	45	48
Irritability	3	31	23	17
Apathy	2	2	2	1

Depression

Thirty-one patients were recorded as being depressed at the time of discharge from hospital; at the six-month follow-up the number had risen to 60. This figure remained remarkably constant throughout the entire follow-up period with only a slight drop at two years. In view of the high incidence of depression we sought to establish how many patients might have been depressed before their accident, and the figure we arrived at was 31. Thus it appeared that most, if not all, of the patients who were depressed in the immediate postaccident phase had already been depressed prior to their injury. It turned out that three patients had been receiving psychiatric treatment immediately before their accidents and seven had made suicidal attempts within the preceding year. It was as a result of a suicidal attempt that one of them was admitted to the study. These figures on depression seem to us to be surprisingly high, and in Table 8.4 we have recorded the numbers of patients with depression during follow-up who had a history of depression at some time prior to their accidents. Depression was seen more commonly in the older age groups. In Table 8.5 we show the mean ages of patients, both male and female, with depression at the various follow-up periods and we contrast them with the mean ages of the whole population studied.

Table 8.4.   Depression at follow-up and prior to injury (Newcastle series).

Follow-up interval	No. of cases		Percentage
	Depression at follow-up	Previous history of depression	
6 months	60	15	25
1 year	58	12	21
2 years	56	10	18

No attempt was made to grade the severity of depression for purposes of recording, but in many instances patients were disturbed enough to require psychiatric treatment. Of those who were depressed at the six-month follow-up, 10 were receiving formal psychiatric treatment; at one year the figure was 15, and at two years 12 were under specialist psychiatric supervision. An attempt was made to differentiate reactive depression from psychotic or endogenous depression. Four of the patients at six months, six at one year, and five at two years were thought to have endogenous depressions and all of them were receiving psychiatric treatment. Half of them had been diagnosed as depressive before their accidents.

No consistent pattern of recovery could be identified in those patients suffering from depression after head injury. As noted already, a significant proportion had a previous history of depression; in some patients the postinjury state seemed simply a continuation of a preaccident illness persisting ultimately throughout the entire two-year follow-up period. In other instances, the depression developed as a late consequence and new cases of depression were diagnosed at all the follow-up intervals; even at the two-year follow-up, there were ten patients who had developed depression since the previous assessment. We were unable to identify any particular factors which

Table 8.5.   Relative mean ages (in years) of patients with depression (Newcastle series).

	Patients with depression		All patients	
	Male	Female	Male	Female
Discharge	43.2	54.1	37.7	42.0
6 months	42.4	58.4	37.1	49.2
1 year	43.3	56.7	36.5	47.9
2 years	42.7	58.7	35.7	48.2

might be responsible for the late development of depression after head injury; in some instances there did seem to be extraneous environmental factors that might be relevant, but in many cases it seemed simply that a previous disorder had become recrudescent.

There was a noticeable association between depression and engagement in a claim for compensation. At the six-month follow-up 67 per cent of patients with depression were making claims for compensation, whereas only 17 per cent of those who were not depressed were claiming. At subsequent follow-ups the figures were similar: 66 per cent, as compared with 23 per cent, at one year, and 70 per cent, as compared with 23 per cent, at two years. The basis for the relationship between depression and compensation claims is probably complex. In many instances the depression expressed itself in terms of physical symptoms such as headache and dizziness and it could be argued that the persistence of such symptoms might have prompted an individual to seek compensation in the belief that they were the direct result of the head injury. On the other hand it could be argued that the pursuit of a claim was likely to engender the continuation of symptoms. As will be discussed in Chapter Eleven, it is our belief that the somatic manifestations of depression are often arbitrarily ascribed to the post-concussional syndrome.

Anxiety

Anxiety was the second most common psychiatric disturbance in patients in the series. As in the case of depression, one of the most important factors associated with anxiety was the preaccident personality. In the year prior to injury, 29 patients in the series were thought to have had definite symptoms of anxiety and, at the six-month follow-up, twelve of the 40 patients with anxiety had suffered a similar illness previously. Table 8.6 indicates the numbers of patients with anxiety at the follow-up periods whose previous history was significant. As will be seen, the proportion of those with such a history fell as the follow-up period advanced. The mean age of the patients with anxiety did not differ significantly from that of the population as a whole, but anxiety symptoms were found to be more common in females than in males.

Table 8.6. Postaccident and preaccident anxiety (Newcastle series).

Interval	No. of cases		Percentage
	Anxiety at follow-up	Previous history of anxiety	
6 months	40	12	30
1 year	45	11	24
2 years	48	8	17

There was a wide range in the severity of anxiety symptoms, but in most instances they were mild in degree. Only five patients in the whole study were thought to require psychiatric treatment directly because of them. An example of a severely affected patient was a man whose injury was due to a frightening accident while travelling as a passenger in a car; his anxiety symptoms, which persisted throughout the two-year follow-up period, were so severe that he was unable to leave his own house unaccompanied. Cases of this type are common in clinical practice and specific phobias may be prolonged and difficult to eradicate. Thus the miner injured by a fall of stone may never be able to return underground, or the scaffolder, after a fall, may never be able to resume working at heights.

As in the case of depression, the patterns of recovery of the anxious patients were quite unpredictable and it proved impossible to construct any consistent recovery curves. Symptoms were frequently late in developing and it was often impossible to determine what had triggered them off, particularly when they appeared only long after the accident. Treatment on the whole was unsatisfactory. Claims for compensation were less common amongst the anxious patients than amongst those with depression. Thirty-seven per cent of those with anxiety at six months, 40 per cent at one year and 35 per cent at two years were pursuing claims, whereas at the same follow-up intervals 24 per cent, 29 per cent and 33 per cent respectively of those not suffering from anxiety were claiming.

Again like depression, anxiety symptoms were often mixed up with somatic complaints such as headache or dizziness. Sometimes the anxiety seemed to be the culmination of a long period of physical complaint. In other patients, however, it was the other way round, with anxiety apparently triggering the physical symptoms.

Cognitive and Memory Disorders

A routine assessment of cognitive function and memory was carried out in the Newcastle patients by means of the standard bedside psychometry used by neurologists. Also a simple scoring system was applied that was based on the Roth Hopkins Information Memory Concentration Test (Roth and Hopkins, 1953). Formal psychometric testing was not obligatory. In the Roth Hopkins test, patients are taken through a series of question inventories. The questions in the information test are concerned mainly with orientation. The memory test consists of a series of questions about the individual being tested and about public events, persons and dates. The concentration test requires the patient to recite the months of the year backwards and to count from one to ten forwards and then in reverse. The test was applied to the majority of patients on their discharge from hospital and at each of the follow-up visits.

Forty-five patients on discharge had a score on the Roth Hopkins Test that indicated impairment of intellectual function. Four of them were known to be of low intelligence prior to their injuries; it was concluded, therefore, that 41 patients had suffered impairment as a result of injury. In all of them, the period of post-traumatic amnesia was greater than 12 hours. In 34 of the patients the intellectual impairment was graded as mild, but in the remaining seven it was severe. Also, thirty-eight patients had significant memory defect, which was particularly severe in two. Confabulation was recorded in eight patients at the time of their discharge from hospital.

Tables 8.7 to 8.9 show the numbers of patients with normal intellectual function, mild impairment or severe impairment at each of the three follow-up periods. Each column is broken down in order to relate the status at follow-up to the assessment made at the time of discharge. It can be seen that the Newcastle patients showed similar recovery patterns to those recorded by others. At six months (Table 8.7) half the patients who were mildly impaired on discharge had returned to normal. By two years (Table 8.9) only four patients classed as mildly impaired at discharge had not returned to normal. Of the seven patients with severe intellectual impairment on discharge, six had improved by six months to the level of a mild deficit and one had returned to normality. By two years, a further two had returned to normal and the remaining four showed a mild defect.

Table 8.7. Intellectual status at 6 months follow-up and at discharge (Newcastle series).

	Six-month follow-up				
	Normal	Mild impairment	Severe impairment	Not Tested*	Total
At discharge:					
Normal	292	0	0	28	320
Mild impairment	17	12	0	5	34
Severe impairment	1	6	0	0	7
Not tested	4	5	1	1	11
Total	*314*	*23*	*1*	*34*	*372*

*Two patients were unable to perform the tests due to profound dementia.

Unfortunately not all of the patients were adequately tested for purposes of categorization, but in a few instances this was due to the fact that other disabilities precluded performance of the tests. Thus a patient already referred to in Chapter Six was prevented from undertaking the tests because of a profound speech defect due to bilateral corticobulbar damage. This raises an important point. In a series of this size, it would have been surprising had there been no patients with profound and permanent dementia. Indeed there were two; their failure to appear in the tables is due simply to the fact that they were beyond the range of the tests on which the tables were based.

Many of the patients with cognitive impairment also showed evidence of behavioural change. At the time of discharge from hospital, 13 patients were exhibiting childish or facile behaviour and in one of them it was particularly marked. By the two-year follow-up visit, although the majority had largely recovered cognitive function as judged by the Roth Hopkins Test, eight were still said by relatives to show persistent behavioural abnormality in that they were slightly facile or disinhibited. A few patients showed evidence of aggression and in three of them this trait persisted right to the end of the follow-up period. Relatives commonly commented that a patient was not quite the same as he or she had been before the accident, implying some degree of personality change.

Table 8.8. Intellectual status at one-year follow-up and at time of discharge (Newcastle series).

	One-year follow-up				
	Normal	Mild impairment	Severe impairment	Not tested*	Total
At discharge:					
Normal	279	0	0	41	320
Mild impairment	24	5	0	5	34
Severe impairment	1	6	0	0	7
Not tested	6	2	0	3	11
Total	*310*	*13*	*0*	*49*	*372*

*Two patients were unable to perform the tests due to profound dementia.

Table 8.9. Intellectual status at two-year follow-up and at time of discharge (Newcastle series).

	Two-year follow-up				
	Normal	Mild impairment	Severe impairment	Not Tested*	Total
At discharge:					
Normal	262	0	0	58	320
Mild impairment	20	4	0	10	34
Severe impairment	3	4	0	0	7
Not tested	6	1	0	4	11
Total	*291*	*9*	*0*	*72*	*372*

*Two patients were unable to perform the tests due to profound dementia.

The Newcastle data would thus support the view that cognitive impairment recovers most rapidly within six months after injury, and only gradual improvement can be anticipated thereafter. Nevertheless, the ultimate prognosis for recovery is surprisingly good, particularly in the young.

Case 193 provides a good illustration of the pattern of recovery. He was a 20-year-old male who was admitted to hospital following a road accident. He was in coma for the first 48 hours after admission, but then gradually recovered consciousness and was well enough to be discharged one month later. The period of post-traumatic amnesia was eventually estimated at three and a half weeks. At the time of discharge from hospital he was euphoric and had little insight into his disability. Nevertheless, he was able to score 33 (upper range of mild impairment) on the Roth Hopkins Test. Two months after the accident a formal WAIS was carried out; his verbal IQ was 100, with performance at 77 and a full scale IQ of 89. Six months after the accident he scored 36 on the Roth Hopkins Test, and his WAIS scores were: verbal—103, performance—85 and full scale—98. Two years later he scored 37 on the Roth Hopkins Test; the WAIS scores were: verbal—108, performance—90 and full scale—101. In spite of this remarkably good recovery, he remained slightly childish and disinhibited. His parents indicated that there had been a significant change in his personality since his accident.

Serious personality change is unfortunately a permanent result of injury in a number of patients. Such patients are among the most tragic of all accident victims. Families can often cope to a remarkable extent with physical disability, but severe behavioural abnormality is liable to stretch them beyond endurance, leading frequently, for instance, to marital break-down. A wide range of disordered behaviour is encountered: sudden aggressiveness, sexual aberration and social irresponsibility. Patients with these characteristics are liable ultimately to need institutional care, but it is true to say that we have little accurate information on how many such patients are permanently housed in our mental hospitals.

REFERENCES

Achte, K. A., Hillbom, E. & Aalberg, V. (1969) Psychoses following war brain injuries. *Acta Psychiatrica Scandinavica*, **45**, 1-18.
Adler, A. (1945) Mental symptoms following head injury. *Archives of Neurology & Psychiatry*, **53**, 34-43.
Bastin, C. H. (1930) Traumatic neurosis. *Canadian Medical Association Journal*, **22**, 653-657.
Bond, M. R. (1975) Assessment of the psychosocial outcome after severe head injury. In *Outcome of Severe Damage to the Central Nervous System. Ciba Foundation Symposium No. 34* (New Series). pp. 141-157. Amsterdam: Elsevier — Excerpta Medica — North Holland.

Bowman, K. M., Blau, A. & Reich, R. (1974) Psychiatric state following head injury in adults and children. In *Injuries of the Brain and Spinal Cord and Their Coverings*. 5th Edition. (Ed.) Feiring, E. H. pp. 570-613. New York: Springer.

Braverman, M. & Hacker, F. J. (1965) Post-traumatic hyperirritability. *Psychoanalytical Review*, **55**, 600-614.

Brock, S. (1960) The neuroses following head (brain) injury. In *Injuries of the Brain and Spinal Cord and Their Coverings*. 4th Edition (Ed.) Brock, S. pp. 328-359. London: Cassell.

Brooks, D. N. (1972) Memory and head injury. *Journal of Nervous and Mental Disease*, **155**, 350-355.

Brooks, D. N. (1974) Recognition memory and head injury. *Journal of Neurology, Neurosurgery and Psychiatry*, **37**, 794-801.

Brooks, D. N. (1976) Wechsler memory scale performance and its relationship to brain damage after severe closed head injury, *Journal of Neurology, Neurosurgery and Psychiatry*, **39**, 593-601.

Conkey, R. C. (1938) Psychological changes associated with head injury. *Archives of Psychology*, **33**, No. 232.

Dencker, S. J. (1958) A follow-up of 128 closed head injuries in twins using co-twins as controls. *Acta Psychiatrica et Neurologica*, **33**, Supplement 123.

Dencker, S. J. (1960) Closed head injuries in twins. *Archives of General Psychiatry*, **2**, 569-575.

Dencker, S. J. and Lofving, B. (1958) A psychometric study of identical twins discordant for closed head injury. *Acta Psychiatrica et Neurologica*, **33**, Supplement 122.

Denny-Brown, D. (1945) Disability after closed head injury. *Journal of the American Medical Association*, **127**, 429-436.

Fahy, T. J., Irving, M. H. and Millac, P. (1967) Severe head injuries. *Lancet*, **i**, 475-479.

Fodor, I. E. (1972) Impairment of memory functions after acute head injury. *Journal of Neurology, Neurosurgery and Psychiatry*, **35**, 818-824.

Foster, J. B., Leiguarda, R. & Tilley, P. J. B. (1976) Brain damage in National Hunt jockeys. *Lancet*, **i**, 981-983.

Goldstein, K. (1952) The effect of brain damage on the personality. *Psychiatry*, **15**, 245-260.

Grinker, R. R. & Spiegel, J. (1945) Men under stress. Philadelphia: Blakiston.

Guttmann, E. (1946) Late effects of closed head injuries: psychiatric observations. *Journal of Mental Science*, **92**, 1-18.

Heiskanen, O. & Sipponen, P. (1970) Prognosis of severe brain injury. *Acta Neurologica Scandinavica*, **46**, 343-348.

Hillbom, E. & Jarho, L. (1969) Post-traumatic Korsakov syndrome. In *The Late Effects of Head Injury*. pp. 98-109 (Ed.) Walker, A. E., Caveness, W. F. & Critchley, M., Springfield, Illinois, U.S.A.: C. C. Thomas.

Kozol, H. L. (1945) & Kozol, H. L. (1946) Pre-traumatic personality and psychiatric sequelae of head injury. I — *Archives of Neurology and Psychiatry*, **53**, 358-364. II — *Archives of Neurology and Psychiatry*, **56**, 245-275.

Lewin, W., Marshall, T. F. De C. & Roberts, A. H. (1979) Long-term outcome after severe head injury. *British Medical Journal*, **ii**, 1533-1538.

Lishman, W. A. (1968) Brain damage in relation to psychiatric disability after head injury. *British Journal of Psychiatry*, **114**, 373-410.

Mandleberg, I. A. & Brooks, D. N. (1975) Cognitive recovery after severe head injury. (I) Serial testing on the Wechsler Adult Intelligence Scale. *Journal of Neurology, Neurosurgery and Psychiatry*, **38**, 1121-1126.

Mandleberg, I. A. (1975) Cognitive recovery after severe head injury. (II) Wechsler Adult Intelligence Scale during post-traumatic amnesia. *Journal of Neurology, Neurosurgery and Psychiatry*, **38**, 1127-1132.

Mandleberg, I. A. (1976) Cognitive recovery after severe head injury. (III) W.A.I.S. Verbal and Performance IQ's as a function of post-traumatic amnesia duration and time from injury. *Journal of Neurology, Neurosurgery and Psychiatry*, **39**, 1001-1007.

Mawdsley, C. & Ferguson, F. R. (1963) Neurological disease in boxers. *Lancet*, **ii**, 795-801.

Merskey, H. & Woodforde, J. M. (1972) Psychiatric sequelae of minor head injury. *Brain*, **95**, 521-528.

Miller, H. (1961) Accident neurosis. *British Medical Journal*, **i**, 919-925, 992-998.

Miller, H. (1966) Mental after-effects of head injury. *Proceedings of the Royal Society of Medicine*, **59**, 257-261.

Miller, H. & Stern, G. (1965) The long-term prognosis of severe head injury. *Lancet*, **i**, 225-229.

Ota, Y. (1965) Psychiatric studies on head injury among the Japanese during the peace time. In *The Proceedings of the 8th International Congress of Neurology*. Verlag der Wiener Medizinischen Akamdemie. pp. 283-286.

Ota, Y. (1969) Psychiatric studies on civilian head injuries. In *The Late Effects of Head Injury*. pp. 110-119. (Ed.) Walker, A. E., Caveness, W. F. & Critchley, M. pp. 110-119. Springfield, Illinois, U.S.A.: C. C. Thomas.

Roche, P. Q. (1960) The dynamics of neurosis following trauma. *Diseases of the Nervous System,* **21,** 100-110.

Roth, M. & Hopkins, B. (1953) Psychological test performance in patients over sixty. *Journal of Mental Science,* **99,** 439-450.

Ruesch, J. (1944) Intellectual impairment in head injury. *American Journal of Psychiatry,* **100,** 480-496.

Ruesch, J. & Bowman, K. M. (1945) Prolonged post-traumatic syndromes following head injury. *American Journal of Psychiatry,* **102,** 145-163.

Russell, W. R. (1968) The traumatic amnesias. *International Journal of Neurology,* **7,** 55-59.

Russell, W. R. & Smith, A. (1961) Post-traumatic amnesia in closed head injury. *Archives of Neurology,* **5,** 426-429.

Symonds, C. P. & Russell, W. R. (1943) Accidental head injury. Prognosis in service patients. *Lancet,* **i,** 7-10.

Tooth, G. (1947) On the use of mental tests for the measurement of disability after head injury. *Journal of Neurology, Neurosurgery and Psychiatry,* **10,** 1-11.

Vigouroux, P. R., Baurand, C., Choux, M. & Guillermain, P. (1972) Etat actuel des aspects sèquellaires graves dans les traumatismes craniens de l'adulte. *Neuro-Chirurgie,* **18,** (Supplement 2).

CHAPTER NINE

Post-traumatic Headache

Headache is undoubtedly the most common of all the sequelae of head injury. It causes protracted distress and incapacity in many of its victims and it taxes the resourcefulness and sometimes the patience of their medical attendants. Most individuals have a natural concern for the well-being of their heads, surpassed only by that reserved for their heart and bowels. In the context of head injury, persistent headache often arouses anxiety about the possibility of pressure, blood clot, or some other less readily conceptualized source of malignity to the brain.

Post-traumatic headache is frequently associated with dizziness, irritability, failure of concentration and intolerance of alcohol. This constellation of symptoms is subsumed under the heading of 'postconcussional syndrome', but headache is undoubtedly the most consistent and troublesome feature. The concept of the postconcussional syndrome is a useful one but it runs the risk of implying, probably erroneously, a single pathogenetic mechanism for all its components. In a later chapter we shall consider the postconcussional syndrome as a whole, but here we are concerned with the single problem of headache.

HISTORICAL REFLECTIONS

The literature on the subject of post-traumatic headache is extensive, but it leaves many questions unanswered. Courville (1953) gives a fascinating account of head injury as recorded in legend and folk tale, and clearly there was early recognition of the phenomenon of post-traumatic headache. It was apparently one Paulus Aeginata (AD 625—690) who first distinguished it from headache due to other causes. Some 600 years later, Theodoric, a contemporary of Lanfranc, described a treatment regime for post-traumatic headache. He also drew attention to the fact that head injury could occur without obvious damage to the skull. Thereafter, little of interest was added to the literature until the latter part of the nineteenth century. With the coming of the Industrial Revolution large numbers of people were exposed to the risk of accidents; safety precautions received scant attention and injury rates were high. Apart from the obvious medical implications of these injuries, their social consequences in terms of loss of work and earnings began to impinge on public awareness, and the subject of head injury attracted a new interest. It was recognized that head-injured patients complained of a wide variety of symptoms; Strumpell (1888) and Friedman (1891) were among the first to attempt to study them systematically. The concept of the post-concussional syndrome emerged from these studies, and the pre-eminence of headache as the most constant and persistent sequel to head injury was recognized.

INCIDENCE OF POST-TRAUMATIC HEADACHE

Published figures on the incidence of post-traumatic headache vary widely. Differences in populations studied, in methods of clinical assessment, in duration of follow-up and in many other parameters make this inevitable. Some quoted figures on the incidence of post-traumatic headache are listed in Table 9.1, which illustrates the wide range referred to and also the generally high figures recorded. The conclusion of Knoflach and Scholl (1937) that 'mild headaches occur in every head injury' was based on a study of no fewer than 1000 cases of head injury caused by blunt objects. They

Table 9.1.   The incidence of post-traumatic headache.

Author	Date	Headache percentage
Russell, W. R.	1932	54.5
Borchardt, M. and Ball, E.	1935	39
Penfield, W. and Norcross, N.	1936	28
Knoflach, J. G. and Scholl, R.	1937	100
Rowbotham, G. F.	1941	80
Guttmann, E.	1943	46
Brenner, C. et al	1944	69
Penfield, W. and Shaver, M.	1945	33
Courville, C. B.	1953	94
Caveness, W. and Nielsen, K.	1961	79
Jacobson, S. A.	1963	75
Tubbs, O. N. and Potter, J. M.	1970	41.5

recorded more intense headache in 36.7 per cent of those with clear evidence of cerebral injury and in 51.5 per cent of those with fractures. Rowbotham's (1941) figure of 80 per cent was based on an examination of 500 patients, and the earlier study of Ritchie Russell (1932), showing an incidence of 54.5 per cent, included 200 patients. A cohort of the same size, consisting of unselected cases of head injury admitted to the Accident Service of the Radcliffe Infirmary in Oxford, was studied by Guttmann (1943). This detailed study showed a 46 per cent incidence of headache in patients on admission or when first able to answer questions. During their stay in hospital the figure remained the same, but it had fallen to 21 per cent when patients were assessed at the time of discharge. There was a later rise in the incidence figure to 38 per cent, but it cannot be discerned from the tables whether this was due to relapse or to the late development of headache in some patients not previously afflicted, and this is a matter to which we will return later when the Newcastle figures are examined. Guttmann found a negative correlation between the severity of the injury and the recorded occurrence of headache and he did not think that age was a significant determining factor. Russell (1933) on the other hand found that post-traumatic headache was much more persistent in patients over 50 years of age.

All the studies quoted so far were carried out on a retrospective basis and were subject to the well-known disadvantages of this method. The study conducted in Boston (Brenner et al, 1944) was designed to be prospective. It included 200 patients admitted to hospital with head injury, 69 per cent of whom had headache in the early stages. A more recent prospective study (Tubbs and Potter, 1970) was concerned with a rather similar group of patients and 41.5 per cent of them were found to have headache during the period in hospital. The Newcastle study produced a figure between these two. In 52.4 per cent of our patients headache was recorded at some time between injury and discharge from hospital (Table 9.2).

Table 9.2. Incidence of headache at different time intervals (Newcastle series).

	Patients with headache		Total patients assessed
	No.	(%)	
During hospitalization	195	52.4	372
On discharge	135	36	372
At six-month follow-up	91	27	338
At one-year follow-up	58	18	323
At two-year follow-up	72	24	300

It would seem a fair generalization to say that headache is not an invariable feature in patients admitted to hospital following head injury, but occurs in about half of them. Unfortunately, no figures are available on the incidence of headache after head injuries not resulting in admission to hospital. In this context we should bear in mind the high incidence of headache in the normal population, regardless of head injury. We should also recognize that the statements on incidence in the foregoing paragraphs tell us nothing of severity or of the incapacity that may result from headache.

Turning to the question of headaches persisting after discharge from hospital, reliable figures are somewhat sparse. We have already referred to the interesting finding of Guttmann (1943) that the number of patients complaining of headache almost doubled during the period immediately after discharge, although by three months it had reverted to the 21 per cent recorded at the time of discharge. Although Brenner et al (1944) showed no such striking increase in incidence in the postdischarge period, six per cent of their patients did develop headache after leaving hospital. Caveness (1966) assessed a group of Korean war veterans who had suffered open or closed head injuries some years previously. He found that no fewer than 80 per cent had a complaint of headache, but he contrasted this figure with a series of uninjured controls, 40 per cent of whom also had headache.

Table 9.2 shows the number of patients in the Newcastle series complaining of headache at different intervals after discharge from hospital. In the first year after injury the incidence gradually fell, but a point of interest was that the numbers rose considerably thereafter, so that at the two-year follow-up the figure was almost as high as at the end of six months.

CLINICAL FEATURES OF POST-TRAUMATIC HEADACHE

One of the most striking features of post-traumatic headache is its variability in site, character, temporal pattern and severity. Characteristically it is intermittent, though Russell (1933) emphasized its continuous nature. Headaches may last for minutes, hours or days and are often described as steady, throbbing, aching, burning or pressing. Although usually generalized, they are sometimes sharply localized and, not infrequently, patients describe sudden severe twinges of pain in a particular area of the scalp. Effort, fatigue, emotional upset or change in posture are often described as precipitating factors, and bright lights and noise are frequent aggravators. Response to rest, quiet and analgesics is highly variable. Curiously enough, these wide variations in the character of post-traumatic headache are encountered both in the early postinjury cases and also in the more chronic persistent ones.

AETIOLOGY OF POST-TRAUMATIC HEADACHE

As is the case with so many of the symptoms that follow head injury, the exact pathogenesis of post-traumatic headache is a matter of controversy. There have been two main schools of thought. One has postulated purely organic mechanisms whilst the other has regarded the disorder as functional. In between these extremes there have been those like Sir Charles Symonds (1970) who have believed that a variety of different mechanisms may operate, and that even in the same patient both organic and functional elements may be present.

In considering this question of pathogenesis, it is important to draw a distinction between the early headaches complained of during the days or weeks following injury and the late variety, which may persist for years. In some patients the late headaches seem to be a direct continuation of the early ones but, as we shall discuss later, there is evidence that in some patients headaches may first develop many months after the injury; in such cases it would seem reasonable to suppose the mechanisms to be different.

As regards the headaches that are so common in the early stages after injury, it seems obvious that some at least result from local damage to the scalp or skull. Brenner et al (1944) emphasized an association between the localization of headache and the site of scalp injury. In our own series, less than 5 per cent of patients complained of localized early headache, but the site of headache in these cases corresponded closely to the area of local injury. Taking early headache in general, regardless of localization, the presence or absence of lacerations and contusions did not make a great deal of difference to the level of its incidence. Those with obvious contusions were slightly more prone to headache in the early stages, but the differences were barely significant.

Knoflach and Scholl (1937) thought that patients with demonstrable skull features had an increased incidence of post-traumatic headache, but the figures of Penfield and Shaver (1945) did not support this. Our findings were in accord with those of the latter authors. Skull fractures were demonstrated in 24 per cent of our entire series and amongst those with headache on discharge from hospital there were 27 per cent with fractures. There is thus little in these figures to support a direct association between fracture and headache.

Before leaving the subject of early headache, it is important to recall the occasional occurrence of subarachnoid haemorrhage, subdural haematoma or even bacterial meningitis in the context of head injury. However, these are relatively uncommon and in our own series they made no significant contribution to the headache figures.

In terms of practical management, it is the persisting headaches after head injury that are the major problem. The widespread and enduring uncertainty about their pathogenesis is surely reflected in the number and variety of suggestions that have been made over the years. Many of them have invoked organic mechanisms, but others have inclined towards psychological explanations. The latter have extended from a charitable concept of 'post-traumatic neurosis' to a somewhat ungenerous belief in the ubiquitousness of commercially inspired malingering. A number of the many suggestions as to pathogenesis are of historical interest only, but others have received continued support over the years and are therefore worthy of mention.

Vasomotor Instability

Bremer et al (1932) regarded vasomotor instability as an important factor in post-traumatic headache. This proposition was discussed at some length by Brenner et al (1944), in the context of earlier observations (Friedman and Brenner, 1944) on the effects of intravenous histamine in patients with localized post-traumatic headache. In 13 out of 20 cases the injection of histamine had provoked a headache identical in character and location to that complained of by the patient. They postulated that, at least in some patients, the pain of post-traumatic headache originates in structures affected by histamine and, quoting Pickering and Hess (1933) and Northfield (1938), they affirmed that the essential element of histamine headache is the painful distension of cerebral arteries. They concluded that the reproduction of localized post-traumatic headache by histamine injection implied the existence of a localized vascular sensitivity resulting from the injury.

Brenner et al (1944) went on to suggest that such a mechanism of post-traumatic headache would account for its association with both physical and emotional influences. They inferred that circulatory changes due to altered posture or physical effort might result in distension of those vessels previously sensitized by trauma, and likewise that arterial distension and consequent pain could result from the circulatory changes induced by emotional reaction. Some support for these theories came from Wolff (1963) who reported that seven per cent of a group of patients with post-traumatic headache had symptoms resulting from distension of extracranial arteries; he based this on observations of the vessels of the scalp. The studies of Haas, Pineda and Lourie (1975) and Vijayan and Dreyfus (1975) also lend support to the view that vascular factors are important in the production of post-traumatic headache.

Against this background it is worth noting that migraine after head injury is uncommon. Friedman (1969) in a study of 8000 patients with migraine found no significant increase in the frequency of attacks following head injury. Nevertheless, attacks of migraine are sometimes provoked by minor head injury and Matthews (1972) has drawn attention to this phenomenon in soccer players. He described a number of them who developed typical migraine attacks immediately after heading a football.

Subdural Adhesions

The notion that subdural adhesions might be responsible for chronic post-traumatic headache was advanced by Penfield and Norcross (1936). They based their theory largely on the experimental production of focal obliterations of the subdural spaces as a result of head injury in the cat. They advocated insufflation of air by lumbar puncture as a treatment for post-traumatic headache, the idea being that adhesions might thereby be broken down, and they reported relief in 60 per cent of their patients. Bearing in mind the natural history of the condition, this figure is not particularly impressive and, as Miller (1968) observed, pneumoencephalography, fortunately no longer part of everyday neurological practice, has a distinct tendency to discourage patients from seeking further attention. Ross and McNaughton (1944) carried out a late review of Penfield's patients and of a group of their own who were similarly treated, but found no evidence that results were any better than in untreated controls.

Cervical Injury

Cyriax (1938) reported that occipital headache radiating to the temples could be induced by the injection of hypotonic saline into the cervical muscles. Two years later Kelly (1940) advocated local injections of cocaine for the relief of such headaches. The idea grew that injury to structures in the neck could be an important cause of post-traumatic headache and additional weight to the theory was added by Jones and Brown (1944), who reported that a high proportion of cases could be relieved by local injection. Jacobson (1963) was another who subscribed to this theory. Whilst there can be no doubt that neck injuries are often sustained at the same time as head injuries, and indeed may go unnoticed because of the effects of the head injury, in our view there has been a tendency to overestimate the contribution of damage to the neck as a cause of the all-too-common chronic form of post-traumatic headache.

Changes in Intracranial Pressure

Both raised and lowered intracranial pressure have been adduced at one time or other as causes of post-traumatic headache. Ritchie Russell (1934) favoured the former. McConnell (1953) held the view that headache was due to localized subdural effusions and he claimed relief of symptoms in 65 patients on whom he had operated and removed collections of subdural fluid, which he found to have a raised protein content. Traumatic rupture of the arachnoid has been suggested by Ingebrigtsen (1969) as the source of these subdural effusions, but their evacuation never became popular as a neurosurgical procedure. Nowadays there is not much support for the idea that they are a significant cause of post-traumatic headache.

A reduction of intracranial pressure might seem a plausible explanation for the occurrence of post-traumatic headache by analogy with the not uncommon lumbar puncture headache believed by most to be due to the leakage of cerebrospinal fluid through a breach in the dura. This process can certainly occur in patients with persistent cerebrospinal fluid rhinorrhoea following head injury, but the idea of a spontaneous low pressure syndrome as a cause of chronic headache (Wolff, 1963) is unattractive.

Local Scalp Injury

We have already referred to the possible role of local injury to the scalp in the pathogenesis of early post-traumatic headache, and have quoted Denny-Brown (1942) and Brenner et al (1944), who found a relationship between the localization of post-traumatic headache and the site of the original injury in a number of patients. It has been suggested that scars developing in the soft tissues of the scalp may produce neuralgic type headaches as a result of the entrapment of branches of sensory nerves (Friedman, 1969). Such headaches are often said to be aggravated by pressure or by exposure to cold.

Sustained Muscle Contraction

Many post-traumatic headaches are indistinguishable in their clinical character-istics from the headaches so often encountered in everyday practice where there is no history of injury and where the label of 'tension headache' is conveniently applied. The pattern must be familiar to all: the tight bands around the head, the feelings of pressure on top of the head and the pains coming up the back of the neck, over the occiput and forward to the temporal or frontal regions. Friedman (1969) believes in the concept of tension headache and he discusses ways in which trauma may lead to sustained muscle contraction and consequent headache. However, because of their similarity to non-traumatic tension headaches, many of which are regarded as psychogenic, the question obviously arises as to the possible role of psychological factors in the production of post-traumatic headaches. This question naturally leads us, albeit with trepidation, into an area of considerable controversy.

Psychological Factors

The debate continues as to the relative importance of organic and psychological factors in the causation of late post-traumatic headache. It is unlikely that the problem will be resolved until we acquire a better understanding of the physiological mechanisms involved in the production of so-called 'functional symptoms'. We cannot explain the non-traumatic headaches, often so appropriately referred to by patients as 'ordinary', which afflict a high proportion of the population. How much more complex the problem when our conjecture has to encompass the additional factor of a head injury, which theoretically could influence a headache reaction in so many different ways. The symbolic significance of the head is sometimes emphasized by those seeking to elaborate a psychodynamic theory. In simpler terms it seems reasonable to suppose that the fright and shock of an accident (perhaps one involving fatality), the worry over possible damage to the brain, the fear of unknown complications, the depression that may follow unhappy events, the stress and perplexity evoked by seemingly interminable legal procedures, not to mention the stimulus of possible financial advantage, may all potentially have a role in triggering this curious propensity to headache that is one of the burdens of mankind.

Most authorities on the subject of post-traumatic headache offer the view that both psychological and organic factors may play a part in their causation, but many seem to emphasize the former with rather more conviction than the latter. Mapother (1937) stressed the psychiatric aspects of post head injury symptoms but nevertheless believed that some of them, though often considered to be psychogenic, were due to subtle brain damage. Lewis (1942) compared a group of patients suffering from the post-concussional syndrome with a group of psychoneurotic patients and could find no factors which clearly distinguished the groups, either in symptomatology or in previous personality. What comes through, from a good many studies, is that post-traumatic headache is common in patients who have previously suffered from psychiatric disorders, in those of low intelligence and in those with hypochondriasis or with inadequate or psychoneurotic personalities (Adler, 1945; Kozol, 1945; Gurdjian and Webster, 1958; Walker and Jablon, 1959; Miller, 1968).

Guttmann (1943), like so many of the authorities quoted, conceded that both physical and psychological factors were contributory, but he clearly expressed the view that the psychological ones were more important. Kay, Kerr and Lassman (1971), whilst conceding the relevance of psychological and social factors, found evidence from a study of 474 patients with head injury that physical causes of headache operated in a number of patients. They based their conclusion largely on the fact that disorders of the special senses were significantly more common in patients with postconcussional symptoms than in those without.

Consideration of the psychological aspects of post-traumatic headache brings us to the difficult question of compensation and its relationship to postinjury symptoms in the medicolegal setting. How often is the complaint of headache after head injury no more than a fabrication or, in other words, how often are we confronted with a conscious malingerer? Opinions differ. It should perhaps be remembered that, quite apart from compensation issues, physicians vary in the extent to which they credit or comprehend the reality of functional symptoms. Although it has been recognized since the Industrial Revolution that compensation for injury creates opportunities for malingering, it was Miller (1961) who in recent times most strongly emphasized the role of conscious simulation in the production of post-traumatic symptoms where questions of compensation arise. He showed that, in a significant number of injury cases, post-traumatic symptoms, most commonly headache, improved after settlement of compensation. He thought the events were related and that they pointed to frank malingering. He drew attention to the fact that post-traumatic symptoms are rare after recreational accidents in contrast to their frequency in those claiming compensation for traffic or industrial injuries. Cook (1972) also found that persisting symptoms and claims for compensation were uncommon after sporting injuries, but commented on the high incidence of persisting headache after injuries involving compensation.

Not everyone would agree with Miller's assessment of the prevalence of conscious malingering. There is a good deal of support for the view that anxiety, depression and some of the other factors already mentioned play a more significant role. However, few would deny that compensation issues do play a part in perpetuating symptoms, in some cases. Perhaps we should give more thought to the adverse effects that the procedures associated with the settlements of compensation claims may have on the natural recovery processes of patients who have been injured. In matters of everyday commerce few of us would claim unwavering objectivity at all times and it is understandable that an individual pursuing compensation, perhaps not of his own volition, may be influenced by repeated enquiry from doctors, lawyers, Trade Union officials and others as to the relationship between his injury and his current state of health and earning ability. For the suggestible, often bewildered litigant it must be extraordinarily difficult to dissociate the pursuit of his claim from his own complex emotions about his accident and those who may have been responsible for it. Most would accept that there is a gap between an understandable propensity to overstate a case and the blatant dishonesty of frank malingering.

THE NEWCASTLE SERIES

By designing our study on a prospective basis we hoped to obtain useful information on the difficult questions relating to post-traumatic headache and its natural history. Before describing our findings, it might be helpful to recall the exact follow-up system that was adopted. On discharge and at each follow-up, patients were subjected to a structured interview so that on each occasion questioning about headache conformed to a standard pattern. Early in the sequence of questions, patients were asked if they had any symptoms and, if a complaint of headache was volunteered at this stage, it was recorded as 'spontaneous'. If symptoms were not forthcoming on this round, the question was repeated and a headache then emerging was designated as 'present with prompting'. Finally, direct enquiry was made about the presence or absence of the symptoms listed in Table 9.3. If a complaint of headache was elicited only in response to direct enquiry, it was designated 'on direct questioning'. The data on headache were analysed separately — for the period of hospitalization, the time of discharge, and at each of the follow-up periods (six months, one year, two years).

Table 9.3. Symptom check list (Newcastle series).

Impaired memory	Alcohol tolerance increased
Impaired concentration	Alcohol tolerance decreased
Emotion absent	Light sensitivity
Depression	Difficulty — seeing
Anxiety	Double vision
Loss of drive	Tinnitus
Incompetence	Difficulty — hearing
Irritability	Difficulty — speaking
Loss of libido	Difficulty — using hands
Impotence/frigidity	Difficulty — using arms
Headache	Difficulty — walking
Dizziness	Difficulty — swallowing
Fatigue	Difficulty with sphincter
Hypersensitivity to noise	Stiff neck
Blackouts	Local tenderness

Scoring: 3 = Volunteered spontaneously; 2 = Elicited with prompting; 1 = Elicited by direct questioning; 0 = Absent.

Early Post-traumatic Headache

Strictly speaking, the category of early post-traumatic headache should include headache recorded both during hospitalization and at the time of discharge from hospital. Of the 372 survivors, 195 (52 per cent) complained of headache at some time during their stay in hospital, but by discharge the figure had fallen to 135 (36 per cent). For purposes of comparing early headache with late, we have focused attention on those recorded at the time of discharge and have disregarded the headaches that had disappeared by that time.

The majority (59 per cent) of patients with post-traumatic headache on discharge complained of it 'spontaneously' (Table 9.4). In 24 per cent, the symptom was volunteered 'with prompting', and in 17 per cent it was elicited only 'on direct questioning'. The age distribution of patients with early headache is shown in Table 9.5. Although the numbers in each age group are quite small, there does appear to be a relatively low incidence in the young and also a fall-off of numbers in the aged. During the working years up to retirement the figures are uniformly high. The highest incidence is in the 25—34 age group, with 52 per cent of all those surviving head injury

Table 9.4. Early headache (on discharge) — type of complaint (Newcastle series).

	No. of cases	(%)
Spontaneous	79	59
With prompting	33	24
On direct questioning	23	17
Total	135	100

complaining of headache at the time of discharge from hospital. Looking at the sex distribution (Table 9.6), and taking all ages together, 44 per cent of women in contrast to 33 per cent of men complained of headache on discharge from hospital. Our figures did not show any association between the occurrence of headache and the type of accident or the particular part of the head injured. Nor was there any association between proneness to headache and social class. In Table 9.7 we have attempted to

Table 9.5. Early headache (on discharge) — age incidence (Newcastle series).

Age (years)	Headache		No headache		Total
	No.	(%)	No.	(%)	
10—14	3	21	11	79	14
15—24	46	36	82	64	128
25—34	23	52	21	48	44
35—44	19	45	23	55	42
45—54	15	44	19	56	34
55—64	16	37	27	63	43
65—74	8	32	17	68	25
75—84	2	13	13	87	15
85 +	3	11	24	89	27
Total	135	36	237	64	372

relate the presence or absence of early headache to the severity of the head injury (as measured by the duration of post-traumatic amnesia). There was a higher incidence of headache in patients with less severe injuries than in those with more severe injuries (with post-traumatic amnesia in excess of one hour).

In Table 9.8, the presence or absence of headache on discharge is related to four other common post-traumatic symptoms: depression, impairment of concentration, anxiety, and dizziness. It is immediately apparent that there is a higher incidence of all of these symptoms in patients with headache than in those without. The association is particularly strong in the case of dizziness, which was complained of by no fewer than 41 per cent of those with headache. In contrast, only seven per cent of patients in the 'no headache' group complained of dizziness. Although not nearly as frequent as dizziness, depression was also much more common in the 'headache' group.

Table 9.6. Early headache (on discharge) — sex incidence (Newcastle series).

	Headache		No headache		Total
	No.	(%)	No.	(%)	
Male	88	33	176	67	264
Female	47	44	61	56	108
Total	*135*	*36*	*237*	*64*	*372*

Persisting Post-traumatic Headache

We have already seen that a lower percentage of patients complained of headache at times of follow-up than during hospitalization or at discharge (Table 9.2). Indeed the proportion with headache at each of the three follow-up periods was fairly constant, representing approximately a quarter of those available for examination. The age and sex distributions of those with and without headache at each of the follow-up intervals are compared in Tables 9.9 to 9.14.

Examination of the prevalence of headache in various age-groups at each follow-up period shows a consistent pattern. Apart from a few odd percentages in the very young and the very old where numbers are small, the curves show a fairly smooth rise and fall with age, with the highest percentage figures in the 45- to 64-years age range. Although the maximum incidence of head injury is in the young, the phenomenon of post-traumatic headache is most frequently encountered in the middle-age to late-middle-age class.

Table 9.7. Early headache (on discharge) — in relation to post-traumatic amnesia (Newcastle series).

Post-traumatic amnesia	Headache		No headache		Total
	No.	(%)	No.	(%)	
Less than 1 hour	76	41	109	59	185
More than 1 hour	44	30	101	70	145
Undetermined	15		27		42
Total	*135*		*237*		*372*

The pattern as regards sex distribution is not quite so consistent. At the six-month follow-up, the percentages of men and women complaining of headache were exactly the same (Table 9.12). By the end of a year the percentage of males complaining of headache had dropped to 15 (Table 9.13), and at two years this figure had made a scarcely significant rise to 18 per cent (Table 9.14). In women, there was no comparable

Table 9.8. Early headache (on discharge) — in relation to other symptoms (Newcastle series).

	Headache (n = 135)		No headache (n = 237)		All patients (n = 372)	
	No.	(%)	No.	(%)	No.	(%)
Depression	24	18	7	3	31	8
Impaired concentration	10	7	4	2	14	4
Anxiety	18	13	12	5	30	8
Dizziness	55	41	17	7	72	19

Table 9.9. Headache at six-month follow-up — age incidence (Newcastle series).

Age (years)	Headache No.	Headache (%)	No headache No.	No headache (%)	Total
10—14	3	23	10	77	13
15—24	27	24	86	76	113
25—34	10	24	31	76	41
35—44	12	30	28	70	40
45—54	13	38	21	62	34
55—64	16	37	27	63	43
65—74	6	25	18	75	24
75—84	1	7	14	93	15
85 +	3	20	12	80	15
Total	*91*	*27*	*247*	*73*	*338*

Table 9.10. Headache at one-year follow-up — age incidence (Newcastle series).

Age (years)	Headache No.	Headache (%)	No headache No.	No headache (%)	Total
10—14	2	15	11	85	13
15—24	15	13	97	87	112
25—34	7	18	31	82	38
35—44	8	21	30	79	38
45—54	8	24	25	76	33
55—64	12	29	30	71	42
65—74	4	18	18	82	22
75—84	1	8	12	92	13
85 +	1	8	11	92	12
Total	*58*	*18*	*265*	*82*	*323*

Table 9.11. Headache at two-year follow-up — age incidence (Newcastle series).

Age (years)	Headache No.	Headache (%)	No headache No.	No headache (%)	Total
10—14	4	36	7	64	11
15—24	13	14	93	86	108
25—34	6	17	30	83	36
35—44	6	17	30	83	36
45—54	12	40	18	60	30
55—64	15	38	25	62	40
65—74	6	29	15	71	21
75—84	2	20	8	80	10
85 +	6	75	2	25	8
Total	*72*	*24*	*228*	*76*	*300*

Table 9.12. Headache at six-month follow-up — sex incidence (Newcastle series).

	Headache		No headache		Total
	No.	(%)	No.	(%)	
Male	64	27	173	73	237
Female	27	27	74	73	101
Total	91	27	247	73	338

drop between six months and a year: the reduction in this interval was only three per cent. However, a slight change occurred at the two-year follow-up at which time the percentage of women complaining of persisting post-traumatic headache had risen to 37. The overall figures would thus suggest that late headache is rather more common in women than in men and that in both sexes it is the 45- to 64-years age group that is most at risk.

We have examined our data to see if there is any relationship between the occurrence of headache at the various follow-up periods and the presence or absence of fracture at the time of the accident (Table 9.15). Out of the whole population of patients who survived the initial head injury, 24 per cent were shown to have a skull fracture. In the group of patients complaining of headache at the time of discharge, 26 per cent had had a skull fracture — a figure very comparable to that for the whole

Table 9.13. Headache at one-year follow-up — sex incidence (Newcastle series).

	Headache		No headache		Total
	No.	(%)	No.	(%)	
Male	35	15	191	85	226
Female	23	24	73	76	97
Total	58	18	265	82	323

group. At all the subsequent follow-up periods, those with headache showed a higher-than-expected incidence of skull fracture. The highest figure was at the six-month follow-up, when 37 per cent of the 91 patients with headache were found to have had fractures. This figure differs significantly from that for the whole group ($P<0.05$). We have also correlated the presence or absence of headache at the follow-up periods with the severity of injury as measured by post-traumatic amnesia. The proportion of patients with persisting headaches and a PTA of less than an hour remains relatively constant throughout the follow-up period (Table 9.16). The inverse relationship between severity of head injury and incidence of headache that was noted in relation to early headache (Table 9.7) is confirmed at all stages of follow-up.

Table 9.14. Headache at two-year follow-up — sex incidence (Newcastle series).

	Headache		No headache		Total
	No.	(%)	No.	(%)	
Male	39	18	172	82	211
Female	33	37	56	63	89
Total	72	24	228	76	300

Table 9.15. Persisting headache and presence or absence of skull fracture (Newcastle series).

	Skull fracture		No skull fracture		X-ray omitted		Total
	No.	(%)	No.	(%)	No.	(%)	
Total patients	88	24	274	74	10	2	372
Headache on discharge	35	26	95	70	5	4	135
Headache at 6-month follow-up	34	37	56	62	1	1	91
Headache at 1-year follow-up	18	31	39	67	1	2	58
Headache at 2-year follow-up	26	36	45	63	1	1	72

A correlation between headache and other postconcussional symptoms, particularly dizziness and depression, has already been noted in the time-of-discharge data (Table 9.8). In Tables 9.17 to 9.19 we make the same analysis for the six-month, one-year and two-year follow-up data and again show that those with headache have a high incidence throughout follow-up of the common postconcussional symptoms which will be discussed further in a later chapter. Dizziness and depression are again prominent, particularly at the six-month and two-year follow-up examinations.

Table 9.16. Persisting headache and duration of post-traumatic amnesia (Newcastle series).

	PTA < 1 hour		PTA > 1 hour		PTA undetermined		Total
	No.	(%)	No.	(%)	No.	(%)	
Total patients	185	50	145	39	42	11	372
Headache on discharge	76	56	44	33	15	11	135
Headache at 6-month follow-up	63	69	28	31	0		91
Headache at 1-year follow-up	38	66	20	34	0		58
Headache at 2-year follow-up	44	61	28	39	0		72

A high proportion of patients in the series became involved in compensation claims. At each follow-up visit they were specifically asked whether or not proceedings had been instituted. At six months 26 per cent of the whole group had done so, at one year 31 per cent and at two years 33 per cent. In the case of those complaining of headache, the proportion seeking compensation was somewhat higher — 48 per cent at six months, 38 per cent at one year and the same at two years.

Table 9.17. Headache at six-month follow-up — in relation to other symptoms (Newcastle series).

	Headache (n = 91)		No headache (n = 247)		All patients (n = 338)	
	No.	(%)	No.	(%)	No.	(%)
Depression	24	26	36	15	60	18
Impaired concentration	11	12	10	4	21	6
Anxiety	18	20	22	9	40	12
Dizziness	44	48	30	12	74	22

Table 9.18. Headache at 1-year follow-up — in relation to other symptoms (Newcastle series).

	Headache (n = 58)		No headache (n = 265)		All patients (n = 323)	
	No.	(%)	No.	(%)	No.	(%)
Depression	15	26	43	16	58	18
Impaired concentration	15	26	17	6	32	10
Anxiety	15	26	30	11	45	14
Dizziness	16	28	29	11	45	14

We have previously described in some detail the methods used for enquiring about symptoms at the follow-up interviews, and have indicated that almost 60 per cent of those patients complaining of headache at the time of discharge volunteered the symptom spontaneously (Table 9.4). It is notable that the level of spontaneity falls off strikingly at each successive follow-up period, until at two years only eight per cent of those with headache complained of it without prompting (Table 9.20).

Table 9.19. Headache at 2-year follow-up — in relation to other symptoms (Newcastle series).

	Headache (n = 72)		No headache (n = 228)		All patients (n = 300)	
	No.	(%)	No.	(%)	No.	(%)
Depression	20	28	36	16	56	19
Impaired concentration	15	21	18	8	33	11
Anxiety	16	22	32	14	48	16
Dizziness	27	38	27	12	54	18

In presenting the data on headache in the follow-up period, we have attempted to make a contrast between the 'early' headache complained of at the time of discharge and the 'persisting' headache recorded at the various follow-up intervals. The group of patients with 'early' headache has therefore been compared with the group suffering from 'persisting' headache, accepting, of course, that there was bound to be an overlap between the two. Apart from a lower incidence of depression in the 'early' group and a greater tendency for the complaint of headache to be offered spontaneously, our comparison between the groups has failed to show any very striking differences. However, when we trace the headache history of individual patients throughout the entire follow-up period from the time of discharge from hospital some interesting facts emerge.

Table 9.20. Type of complaint of patients with headache at follow-up intervals (Newcastle series).

	Discharge		6 months		1 year		2 years	
	No.	(%)	No.	(%)	No.	(%)	No.	(%)
Spontaneous	79	59	30	33	15	26	6	8
With prompting	33	24	14	15	7	12	44	61
On direct questioning	23	17	47	52	36	62	22	31
Total	135		91		58		72	

The Natural History of Post-traumatic Headache

We have already examined the figures for the numbers of patients complaining of headache at the various follow-up periods (Table 9.2). These figures are reproduced in graphic form in Figure 9.1, which illustrates the progressive fall in numbers with the passage of time, except for a slight upturn at the end of the follow-up period. It would be reasonable to conclude that these figures are illustrating the gradual recovery of a proportion of patients, together with a somewhat surprising late relapse of a small number of them. If we trace the headache patterns in individual patients we find that this conclusion is erroneous. In fact, there was a far higher recovery rate than Figure 9.1 would suggest and, as is illustrated in Figure 9.2, little over half the patients who complained of headache at the follow-up interviews had been suffering from it at the time of discharge. In other words, a substantial proportion of those complaining of headache at follow-up had been free of headache at the time of discharge and had acquired their headaches in the follow-up period. We shall refer to these headaches as 'late acquired' and designate those which were a continuation of a headache on discharge as 'persisting'. It should be noted that the 'persisting' group does contain a small number where there had been recovery at twelve months but relapse by the end of two years.

The two headache populations thus identified in the follow-up period are roughly the same size. If we examine their age and sex distributions we find that they do not differ significantly; likewise the severity of the original head injuries, as measured by the means of the periods of post-traumatic amnesia, is similar in the two groups. The distribution of social classes is the same in each, as is the incidence of skull fracture, and the numbers are very similar in the two groups as regards the types of accident. groups.

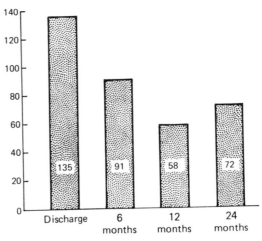

Figure 9.1. Numbers of patients with headache on discharge and at follow-up (Newcastle series).

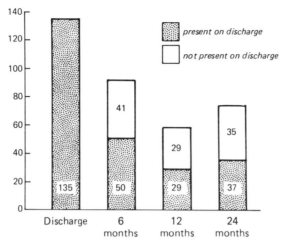

Figure 9.2. Headaches during follow-up according to presence or absence on discharge (Newcastle series).

Whilst the 'late acquired' and 'persisting' headache groups are thus very similar as regards most of their characteristics, there are one or two striking differences. We have already seen that the pursuit of compensation claims is more common amongst those with headache in the follow-up period than amongst those without. When we look at this feature specifically in relation to the headache groups we have now defined, we find that compensation claims are associated with the 'late acquired' group much more than with the 'persisting' group. No less than 83 per cent of patients with 'late acquired' headache at six months were initiating compensation claims, as compared with 20 per cent in the 'persisting' group. The respective figures for the two groups at one year were 62 per cent and 14 per cent, and at two years they were 57 per cent and 19 per cent (Table 9.21). Various theoretical interpretations can be put on these figures, but they make the case for an organic relationship between the injury and the 'late acquired' headache difficult to sustain.

The other important difference between the 'late acquired' and 'persisting' headache groups is that the former show a higher incidence of depression. The difference is very striking in the analysis at the six-month follow-up, when 44 per cent

Table 9.21. Percentage of patients with 'persisting' and 'late acquired' headache pursuing compensation claims (Newcastle series).

Claims pending	'Persisting' (%)	'Late acquired' (%)
At six months	20	83
At one year	14	62
At two years	19	57

of those with 'late acquired' headache were suffering from depression as opposed to 12 per cent of those with 'persisting' headache (Table 9.22). The figures were rather less striking at the later follow-up periods. At one year 31 per cent of the 'late acquired' group were depressed as opposed to 21 per cent of the 'persisting' group. At two years the figures were 34 per cent and 22 per cent respectively. The study thus confirms the widely accepted clinical impression of a relationship between depression and post-traumatic headache and it illustrates the particular association with the 'late acquired' type of headache, revealed by the prospective analysis. We have long held the view that depression is an important cause of post-traumatic headache rather than the other way round.

The role of depression in the causation of post-traumatic headache is illustrated by the following case histories.

Table 9.22. Percentage of patients with 'persisting' and 'late acquired' headache suffering from depression (Newcastle series).

Depression	'Persisting' (%)	'Late acquired' (%)
At six months	12	44
At one year	21	31
At two years	22	34

Case 227. A 70-year-old female suffered a blow to the left frontal region when the bus in which she was travelling was involved in an accident. Her head injury was minor with no skull fracture, no loss of consciousness and no post-traumatic amnesia. The only significant injury was a severe laceration of the left leg. She was detained in hospital for a few days and at the time of discharge her sole complaint was of soreness of the leg. Six months later she was still symptom-free, apart from persisting leg pain, but at the one-year follow-up the situation had changed. She had developed symptoms of a moderately severe depression, for which she was under treatment by her family doctor, and she complained of constant headache. Her persisting leg pain was the basis of a claim for compensation. This was settled shortly before her final two-year follow-up, when both her headache and depression were better although neither was fully recovered.

It was thought that the depression had been largely due to the persisting pain in her leg and the consequent restriction of her activity; her headache was regarded as a symptom of the depression.

Case 283. This case also illustrates the development of depression with associated headache as a result of bodily injuries. A 64-year-old female was knocked down by a motor car and suffered a closed head injury with loss of consciousness post-traumatic amnesia of 30 minutes duration, but no skull fracture. She had a severe fracture of her pelvis. During her stay in hospital and at the time of her discharge she complained of positional vertigo, which was accompanied by nystagmus in all directions of gaze. She denied headache. At the six-month follow-up she still had positional vertigo and nystagmus and she complained of severe pain in her pelvis on walking. At the one-year follow-up, although still complaining of dizziness, positional nystagmus could not be elicited. Severe pelvic pain persisted. At the two-year follow-up the position had deteriorated. She complained that her dizziness was more pronounced, although again there was no positional nystagmus. Pains in the pelvic region persisted; in addition, she now complained of severe headaches and of increasing depression, which she attributed to the marked restriction in her activity. Three months before her final visit to the clinic, she had been awarded £1000 in compensation for loss of earnings but this did not seem to influence her symptomatology in any way.

As in the previous case, we assumed that this patient suffered from functional headaches as part of a depression resulting from both the psychological and physical trauma of a road accident and its consequences.

Case 101. This illustrates the not uncommon situation where the circumstances of the accident and its recollection have a more powerful effect on the patient than do the physical injuries, and where psychological breakdown may be precipitated by re-exposure to the circumstance in which the accident occurred. A 38-year-old coalminer suffered a left parietal injury whilst working underground. Loss of consciousness was brief and the period of post-traumatic amnesia was assessed at only five minutes. There was no skull fracture. The patient was fully recovered and asymptomatic on discharge from hospital, but at the six-month follow-up he complained of persisting headaches at the site of injury. He stated that these headaches had first developed on return to work, four weeks after discharge from hospital, and he recalled that he developed severe symptoms of anxiety on returning to the coal face and had to be brought out of the mine. Thereafter he experienced continuing symptoms of anxiety and depression together with severe headache. He had been awarded a five per cent disability pension prior to his six-month follow-up visit and was making no other claims for compensation. At the one-year follow-up he was still complaining of recurring headache, but symptoms of anxiety and depression had improved and he had been able to return to work. By the two-year follow-up he had completely recovered except for occasional headaches.

The above three patients exemplify the association between post-traumatic depression and late acquired post-traumatic headache. They all had previously stable personalities with no symptoms of psychiatric illness. All of them continued to complain of severe headache after compensation claims or disability assessments had been settled; they illustrate the widely accepted fact that symptoms do not necessarily subside when the financial implications are resolved.

In these cases we doubt that matters of compensation were of importance in relation to the headaches. However, attention has been drawn to a statistical relationship between late acquired post-traumatic headache and the pursuit of compensation claims. We have already expressed the view that the psychodynamics of this association are complex and that to assume deliberate fabrication or frank malingering is to oversimplify. Nevertheless, we would certainly not deny that indisputable cases of malingering are encountered and in the whole series there two patients who were thought to be attempting deliberately to mislead the examiner on repeated occasions, in the hope of advancing their compensation claims. Both patients were thought to be simulating loss of taste and smell and both cheerfully denied all ability to detect an ammonia solution, in spite of their tears and obvious signs of fifth nerve stimulation.

Case 35. The final case illustrated the possible relevance of previous psychiatric history to the development of post head injury symptoms, including headache. The patient was a 33-year-old female who suffered a minor head injury when travelling in a bus which was involved in an accident. Loss of consciousness was brief and post-traumatic amnesia was estimated at five minutes. She was asymptomatic on discharge from hospital, but at the six-month follow-up she had a multiplicity of symptoms including headache, difficulty in breathing, anxiety and depression. These symptoms caused major disability and they persisted unabated for the next two years, in spite of psychiatric treatment. The patient had a psychiatric history going back some ten years before her accident. She had complained of frequent blackouts which were not epileptic and she had had many symptoms of anxiety. She had been seen by many psychiatrists over the years and had been regarded as an inadequate person with a neurotic depressive tendency. The pattern of her symptoms following the accident was very similar to that experienced previously, and during both periods she was strikingly unresponsive to psychiatric treatment. After her accident she received a very reasonable compensation payment, but this had no influence on the pattern of her illness.

This patient presented a problem that is all too familiar in clinical practice. The individual with a neurotic personality is ill-equipped to cope with the additional physical and psychological strains resulting from head injury, which exaggerates and perpetuates pre-existing complaints.

SUMMARY

Whilst the case histories that we have quoted illustrate some of the well-recognized patterns of postinjury headache, the variety is infinite and in a great many cases no satisfactory explanation can be found for the persistence of headache. The most important result of our study has been the recognition of 'late acquired' post-traumatic headache, and the fact that this group comprises approximately half of those patients with persistent headache following a head injury. We believe that recognition of this group is important in relation to theories of pathogenesis of post-traumatic headache and have pointed out the particular association between late acquired headache and both depression and claims for compensation. Unfortunately, it is difficult to recognize patients with this type of post-traumatic headache, except in the context of a prospective study, because most of the patients who fall into this category are under the impression that their headache dates from the time of injury, even though the documented evidence is to the contrary.

In conclusion, we would reflect on the fact that our observations on the delayed development of headache are by no means original. We are simply reviving what Charcot in a more poetic age referred to as 'the period of meditation'.

REFERENCES

Adler, A. (1945) Mental symptoms following head injury. *Archives of Neurology and Psychiatry,* **53,** 34-43.
Borchardt, M. & Ball, E. (1935) Headache after injuries to the head and spine. *Archives of Orthaepedics and Mechanical Therapy,* **35,** 227-229.
Bremer, F., Coppez, H., Hicquet, G. & Martin, P. (1932) Le syndrome commotionnel tardif dans les tramatismes fermés due crâne. *Revue due Oto Neuro Opthalmologie,* **10,** 161-224.
Brenner, C., Friedman, A. P., Houston-Merritt, H. & Denny-Brown, D. E. (1944) *Post Traumatic Headache,* **1,** 379-391.
Caveness, W. F. (1966) Post traumatic sequelae. *Head Injury* (Ed.) Caveness, W. F. & Walker, A. E. Chapter 17 Philadelphia and Toronto: J. B. Lippincott.
Caveness, W. & Nielsen, K. (1961) Sequelae of cerebral concussion. *New York State Journal of Medicine,* **61,** 1871-1886.
Cook, J. B. (1972) The post concussional syndrome and factors influencing recovery after minor head injury admitted to hospital. *Scandinavian Journal of Rehabilitation Medicine,* **4,** 27-30.
Courville, C. B. (1953) *Commotio Cerebri.* Los Angeles: San Lucas Press.
Cyriax, J. (1938) Rheumatic headache. *British Medical Journal,* **ii,** 1367-1368.
Denny-Brown, D. (1942) The sequelae of war head injuries. *New England Journal of Medicine,* **227,** 771-779, 813-821.
Friedman, A. P. (1969) The so called post traumatic headache. *The Late Effects of Head Injury* (Ed.) Walker, A. E., Caveness, W. F. & Critchley, M. Chapter 5. Springfield, Illinois, U.S.A.: C. C. Thomas.
Friedman, A. P. & Brenner, C. (1944) Post traumatic and histamine headache. *Archives of Neurology and Psychiatry, Chicago,* **52,** 126-130.
Friedman, M. (1891) Uber eine besondere Form von Folgezustanden nach Gehirnerschutterung under uber den vasomotorischen Symptomenocomplex bei derselben im Allgerneinen. *Archiv fur Psychiatrie,* **23,** 230-238.
Gurdjian, E. S. & Webster, J. C. (1958) Head injuries. In *Mechanisms of Diagnosis and Management.* Chapter 6. Boston: Little Brown.
Guttmann, E. (1943) Post contusional headache. *Lancet,* **i,** 10-12.
Haas, D. C., Pineda, G. S. & Lourie, H. (1975) Juvenile head trauma syndromes and their relationship to migraine. *Archives of Neurology,* **32,** 727-730.
Ingebrigtsen, B. (1969) Arachnoid rupture as cause of the post concussion syndrome. *Acta Neurologica Scandinavica,* **45,** 231-237.
Jacobson, S. A. (1963) *The Post Traumatic Syndrome Following Head Injury.* Springfield, Illinois: C. C. Thomas.
Jones, O. W. Junior and Brown, H. A. (1944) The treatment of post traumatic head pain. *Journal of Nervous and Mental Diseases,* **99,** 668-671.
Kay, D. W. K., Kerr, T. A. & Lassman, L. P. (1971) Brain trauma and the postconcussional syndrome. *Lancet,* **ii,** 1052-1055.
Kelly, M. (1940) Muscular Pain. *Western Australian Clinical Reference,* **1,** 51-53.
Knoflach, J. C. & Scholl, R. (1937) *Archiv fur Klinische Chirurgie,* **190,** 452-522.
Kozol, H. (1945) Pre traumatic personality and psychiatric sequelae of head injury. *Archives of Neurology and Psychiatry,* **53,** 358-364.
Lewis, A. (1942) Discussion on differential diagnosis and treatment of post-contusional states. *Proceedings. Royal Society of Medicine,* **35,** 607-614.

Mapother, E. (1937) Mental symptoms associated with head injury; the psychiatric aspect. *British Medical Journal,* **ii,** 1055-1061.

Matthews, W. B. (1972) Footballers migraine. *British Medical Journal,* **ii,** 326-327.

McConnell, A. A. (1953) On certain sequelae of closed head injuries. The pathological basis of post traumatic syndrome. *Brain,* **76,** 473-484.

Miller, H. (1961) Accident neurosis. *British Medical Journal,* **i,** 919-925, 992-998.

Miller, H. (1968) Post traumatic headache. In *Handbook of Clinical Neurology* (Ed.) Vinken, P. J. & Bruyn, G. W. Volume 5, Chapter 14, pp. 178-184. Amsterdam: North Holland Publishing.

Northfield, D. W. C. (1938) Some observations on headache. *Brain,* **61,** 133-162.

Penfield, W. & Norcross, N. (1936) Subdural traction and post traumatic headache. *Archives of Neurology and Psychiatry,* **36,** 75-94.

Penfield, W. & Shaver, M. (1945) The incidence of traumatic epilepsy and headache after head injury in civil practice. *Research Publications of the Association for Nervous and Mental Disorders,* **24,** 620-634.

Pickering, G. W. & Hess, W. (1933) Observations on the mechanism of headache produced by histamine. *Clinical Science,* **1,** 77-101.

Ross, W. D. & McNaughton, F. L. (1944) Head injury; a study of patients with chronic post traumatic complaints. *Archives of Neurology and Psychiatry, Chicago,* **52,** 255-269.

Rowbotham, G. F. (1941) Complications and sequelae of injuries to the head. *Medical Press,* **205,** 379-384.

Russell, W. R. (1932) Cerebral involvement in head injury: a study based on the examination of two hundred cases. *Brain,* **55,** 549-562.

Russell, W. R. (1933) After-effects of head injuries. *Transactions of the Medical Chirurgical Society of Edinburgh,* **113,** (1933-34), 129-141.

Russell, W. R. (1934) Discussion on intracranial pressure; its clinical and pathological importance. *Proceedings of the Royal Society of Medicine,* **27,** 832-834.

Strumpell, A. (1888) *Uber die traumatischen Neurosen.* Berlin: Gustav Fischer.

Symonds, C. P. (1970) Concussion and contusion of the brain and their sequelae. In *Injuries of the Brain & Spinal Cord* (Ed.) Feiring, E. H. Fifth Edition. Chapter four. New York: Springer Publishing.

Tubbs, O. N. & Potter, J. M. (1970) Early post concussional headache. *Lancet,* **ii,** 128-129.

Vijayan, N. & Dreyfus, P. M. (1975) Post traumatic dysautonomic cephalalgia. *Archives of Neurology,* **32,** 649-652.

Walker, F. & Jablon, S. (1959) A follow up of head injured men of World War II. *Journal of Neurosurgery,* **16,** 600-610.

Wolff, H. G. (1963) *Headache and Other Head Pain.* Second Edition. New York: Oxford University Press.

CHAPTER TEN

Post-traumatic Dizziness

INTRODUCTION

'There can be few physicians so dedicated to their art that they do not experience a slight decline in spirits on learning that their patient's complaint is of giddiness'. Thus Matthews (1963) starts the chapter on giddiness in his delightful book *Practical Neurology*. Dizziness and giddiness must be among the most difficult of all symptoms to unravel and this is particularly so in the context of head injury. Here they are so often mixed up with other symptoms commonly thought, at least in part, to be neurotic. There are a wide variety of odd and often unpleasant sensations in the head to which man is subject, and the problem is compounded by the availability of a wide range of terms to describe them. Whilst some people maintain that words like giddiness, dizziness and vertigo have separate and distinct meanings, others regard them as interchangeable; the Oxford English Dictionary largely supports the latter view. Certainly there are no clear-cut definitions and, as Matthews says, enquiry into what is meant by giddiness is likely to receive the answer that it is 'like what you feel when you feel giddy!' We cannot presume to clarify the issue, and frequently in this chapter we shall quote terms used by other authors without being able to define exactly what they meant.

Dizziness as a sequel to head injury was described in legend and folk tale long before there were any medical writings on the subject. Courville (1953) cited a number of interesting examples from the past, and related that Alexander the Great and Captain Cook were both numbered amongst those who had suffered from traumatic vertigo. In medical literature, Galen was probably the first to refer to vertigo after head injury (Darenberg, 1854). Until the late nineteenth century it was generally believed that vertigo was a manifestation of congestion of the brain and meninges, even though a number of people like John Hall (1679), Shakespeare's brother-in-law, had noted the coexistence of vertigo and deafness in some cases. The credit for first establishing an association between vertigo and disorders of the ear must go to Prosper Ménière (1861), although there now seems little doubt that his original patient did not suffer from the syndrome that bears his name.

Turning to the specific question of trauma in relation to the ear and vestibular system, we find that Risk (1890) described injury to the labyrinth. But, like others of his time, he associated the labyrinth only with acoustic function and made no reference to vestibular symptoms. The early twentieth century literature on head injury and the ear was ably reviewed by Linthicum and Rand (1931). Included in their review was a paper by Halz (Linthicum and Rand, 1931), which described a patient with postural vertigo caused by a gunshot wound. They also referred to a report by Rhese (Linthicum and Rand, 1931) on 45 patients with concussion, many of whom had disturbances of both equilibrium and hearing. Passow (1905), also quoted by Linthicum and Rand, suggested that damage to the inner ear was a common occurrence in severe head injuries, and Stenger (Linthicum and Rand, 1931) described gross pathological and microscopic changes in the inner ear in patients who had died from head injury.

These early writings clearly established an association between head injury and vestibular disorder, both clinical and pathological. In order to understand more modern views on post-traumatic dizziness it is necessary to pick up another thread: namely, the development of our ideas on vestibular physiology and the ways in which it may be studied in the clinical laboratory. The principal character in this story is Robert Bárány, who was not only the first to devise clinical tests of vestibular function, but also demonstrated their value in the diagnosis of intracranial lesions. One of Bárány's major contributions was to recognize that nystagmus may vary, depending on the position of the head and Preber and Silfverskiöld (1957) refer to a Bárány publication of 1910 that describes for the first time the phenomenon of positional nystagmus. His definitive paper (Bárány, 1921), which is generally regarded as the first description of positional nystagmus, included a generous reference to the crucial observation made by his assistant. It reads: 'Dr. Carlefors first noted that the attack appeared when she (the patient) lay on her right side. When she did this there appeared a strong rotatory nystagmus to the right. The attack lasted about thirty seconds and this was accompanied by violent vertigo and nausea. If immediately after the cessation of the symptoms the head was again turned to the right no attack occurred and in order to evoke a new attack in this way the patient had to lie for some time on her back or on her left side'. Bárány subsequently showed that the factor precipitating the vertigo was not the head movement itself, but the change of the position of the head in space. For this reason he attributed it to a disorder of the otoliths. He also made the observation that positional vertigo and positional nystagmus could occur as a result of head injury.

So far we have concentrated on the literature concerning the relationship between the ear and vestibular symptoms in the context of head injury. In addition, there is a substantial literature describing other suggested mechanisms which might account for dizziness following trauma. Among them is the description by Barré (1926) of the 'posterior sympathetic syndrome', which postulates damage to sympathetic nerves around the vertebral arteries. 'Vasomotor disturbances', often of rather doubtful physiological authenticity, have also been supposed to be responsible for post-traumatic dizziness. Perhaps the most substantial literature of all in the field relates to the role of psychoneurosis in the causation of these symptoms. Later in the chapter we will come back to some of these other aetiological theories.

INCIDENCE OF POST-TRAUMATIC DIZZINESS

As with headache, the incidence of post-traumatic dizziness quoted in the literature varies considerably, depending on case selection. In an early review Mygind (1918) found that 24 of a series of 100 patients 'with ordinary fresh lesions of the head' had 'genuine objective vestibular symptoms'. Indeed, he asserted that as many as one-third had suffered a 'traumatic vestibular disease'. Schuster (1927) claimed an incidence of 40 per cent of ear symptoms after head injury, whilst Linthicum and Rand (1931) maintained that practically all cases suffered from some dizziness, and approximately 90 per cent had 'some degree of equilibratory disturbance'. These latter authors assert that only ten per cent actually complain of true rotational vertigo. Other early figures vary from 21 per cent (Russell, 1932) to 57 per cent (Osnato and Gilibertini, 1927) and 60 per cent (Glaser, 1937).

We have referred in other chapters to the important prospective head injury study carried out in Boston by Denny-Brown and his colleagues. In 1945 they published a report on the investigation of post-traumatic dizziness in their group of patients (Friedman, Brenner and Denny-Brown, 1945). The authors quoted an incidence of 50 per cent for 'dizziness' after injury, though they could find only 6 per cent with 'true vertigo'. In the same year, Phillips (1945) noted what he called 'giddiness' in over 30 per cent of all types of head injury, and found true vertigo in half of these. Subsequent studies have confirmed that something like 50 per cent of patients suffering a closed head injury will develop vertigo (Caveness and Nielson, 1961; Jacobson, 1963). The first of these was a study based on 407 people wounded in the Korean war. It is of some considerable interest, as the authors were the first to note the incidence of dizziness in a control group, of whom 17 per cent had symptoms similar to those experienced by the head injury group.

AETIOLOGY OF POST-TRAUMATIC DIZZINESS

Four mechanisms have been mentioned which have been alleged to play a part in the causation of post-traumatic dizziness. Each will be considered in some detail.

Vasomotor Disorders

The idea that 'vasomotor instability' may be an important element in the causation of post head injury symptoms has enjoyed popularity since the subject was first studied. Certainly it has been thought by many to be relevant in the case of post-traumatic dizziness, but this is presumably because of the character of the symptoms that so many patients describe. In the various clinical papers that we have already referred to, there has been less emphasis on true vertigo following head injury than on descriptions of faintness and light-headedness, often in relation to postural change. This tendency for dizziness to be precipitated by postural change was noted particularly by Russell (1932). He commented that post-traumatic dizziness was most commonly precipitated by movements such as standing, which tended to 'lower the intracranial blood-pressure'. This led him to emphasize the possibility of circulatory disturbances. He attributed the slow resolution of symptoms to the fact that maladjustments of intracranial circulation are slow to recover. Symonds (1942) tended to support these views on the relevance of circulatory changes, and suggested that they might in some cases be due to medullary concussion resulting from injury. There is not much experimental evidence to support the theory but Courville (1953), after reviewing the early literature on the subject and adding his own observations not only on clinical histories, but also on pathological studies of fatal cases, concluded that post-concussional symptoms, including headache and confusion as well as dizziness, are produced on the basis of impaired vasomotor control which can no longer adjust satisfactorily to postural change.

There have been a few clinical studies which have sought to examine particularly the vasomotor theory and which have included specific physiological observation. Bennett (1910), in a study of patients suffering from post-traumatic symptoms, noted lability of pulse rate and volume, but this was the only evidence in support of vasomotor disturbance. The Boston group (Friedman, Brenner and Denny-Brown, 1945) examined 11 patients using a tilt table. Eight had postural dizziness or vertigo. All the subjects were tilted from the head-down to the head-up position and examined for evidence of vasomotor abnormality. Any changes noted were mild, and certainly of no greater severity than those found in normal controls. They concluded that there was no evidence for systemic vasomotor instability in the group they examined. Subsequent workers carrying out similar experiments have failed to find much support for the notion of vasomotor instability. Taylor and Bell (1966) and Taylor (1967) thought that they could show changes in cerebral circulation after concussional head injury, but their technique did not give an absolute measure of cerebral blood flow. The consensus now is that vasomotor instability is not a satisfactory explanation for post-traumatic dizziness.

Cervical Spine and Dizziness

That disorders of the neck or cervical spine may be associated with dizziness has been claimed for many years, though this has often been disputed. In 1926, Barré first described his 'posterior sympathetic syndrome' and ascribed it to arthritis of the cervical spine; the syndrome was subsequently extended into a polymorphic clinical picture by Lieou (1928). Extensive reviews of the literature concerning cervical vertigo, cervical nystagmus and the syndrome of Barré may be found in the publications of Gayral and Neuwirth (1954), Jongkees (1969) and Biemond and DeJong (1969). Of these authors, only Gayral and Neuwirth refer to the role of trauma in producing the syndrome. The now-common term 'whiplash' was probably used first by Davis in 1945 to describe the mechanism of neck injuries resulting from head-on collisions. A fuller recognition of the so-called 'cervical syndrome' after such injuries owes much to the work of Jackson (1966) in America, but, with a few exceptions (Ryan and Cope, 1955), the syndrome has attracted less attention in Great Britain. For those interested in the various theories to account for vertigo of cervical origin, we would refer to the review of Compere (1968). He examined 47 patients with post-whiplash injury dizziness, using the technique of electronystagmography (ENG). Fifty-six per cent had an abnormal ENG, and the majority of these showed nystagmus that was precipitated only by rotation or extension of the head. None was found to have nystagmus when the head was placed to the side without rotating the neck, so Compere thought that the neck rotation rather than the head position was the important factor in the production of nystagmus and vertigo. He concluded that positional vertigo after whiplash injury is caused by compression of the vertebral artery against the transverse process of the seventh cervical vertebra when the neck is either rotated or extended, with resulting brain stem ischaemia. The same author went on to study the problem using the technique of rheoencephalography (Compere, 1971), and he claimed to confirm his theory. Changes in blood flow demonstrated by this technique are difficult to interpret because it reflects not only intracranial circulation, but also circulation through the scalp.

Psychological Factors

Dizziness is a significant component of the post-traumatic or postconcussional syndrome: it is in this setting that its psychological aspects have been particularly emphasized in the literature. The post-traumatic syndrome will be discussed as such in a later chapter, but one particular point about it is relevant at this stage. We refer to the fact that within the syndrome a number of differing causal mechanisms may be operating at the same time. It is often difficult to pinpoint the aetiology of an individual symptom after head injury, but when symptoms are combined together into a pattern it may become virtually impossible. Very often we seek refuge in compromise and conclude that the symptom complex is partly organic and partly psychologically induced. This point of view was certainly adopted over 30 years ago by Strauss and Savitsky (1934) and has subsequently attracted support (Schaller, 1939; Caveness, 1966). Schaller attempted to differentiate between what he called a 'post-traumatic psychoneurotic state' (psychoneurosis/hysteria) and a 'post-traumatic concussion state' (concussion/traumatic encephalopathy). He regarded the descriptions of the symptoms themselves as of paramount importance; for instance, he was inclined to equate 'giddiness' with the post-traumatic psychoneurotic state, and 'vertigo' with the post-traumatic concussion state. Silfverskiöld (1969) also referred to the importance of symptoms in differentiating between the two categories. He emphasized the tendency to find objective physical signs in the organic group, and functional and bizarre physical anomalies in the psychological group. We have already referred to the question of psychological factors in the production of post head injury symptoms and to the relevance of compensation issues in Chapter Eight.

Vestibular Factors

Historical Review

We have referred to the work of Robert Bárány and to his description of positional vertigo following head injury. One of the first systematic attempts to demonstrate that post-traumatic dizziness was of vestibular origin was made by Mygind (1918). He examined 142 patients with head injury and found spontaneous rotary nystagmus in 26, although the nystagmus 'in some cases was only discovered by little tricks' such as 'certain movements of the head'. Mygind made the pertinent observation that the vestibular symptoms were often not prominent in the first few days after injury, and rarely cleared quickly once they had developed. Schuster (1927), in a later review of the subject, claimed that such symptoms sometimes persisted indefinitely, though he produced no evidence to support this.

Grove (1928) described the clinical and pathological findings in 42 head-injured patients and concluded that postconcussional vertigo, if of vestibular origin, was characterized by dizziness and nystagmus brought on by movement of the head. Linthicum and Rand (1931) agreed in part with Grove, but thought their findings pointed to mixed central and end-organ damage as the cause of post-traumatic dizziness. Their most constant clinical finding was past-pointing. A few years later Glaser (1937) reviewed his extensive experience of 325 cases of head injury; 60 per cent of them suffered dizziness, but none had what he called true vertigo. He carried out tests of vestibular function on 66 of the patients, both dizzy and non-dizzy, and reported that 40 per cent had evidence of central lesions, 36 per cent had evidence of end-organ lesions and 24 per cent had normal vestibular responses. Nevertheless, he said that only 25 per cent of those with normal responses had no dizziness, and substantial numbers amongst those with alleged central and end-organ lesions likewise had no dizziness. Glaser's figures showed a poor correlation between abnormal vestibular tests and symptoms of dizziness, but it should be noted that he did not include tests for positional nystagmus among his investigations of vestibular function.

Brunner (1940), reviewing the literature up to that date, commented particularly that spontaneous nystagmus is often missed in patients with post-traumatic dizziness unless they are examined after the head has been moved quickly backwards. He was clearly describing positional nystagmus, but he made no reference to it as such and did not quote the work of Bárány. In a fairly extensive study in which he employed caloric testing, Phillips (1945) found, like Glaser (1937), a high incidence of abnormality in head-injured patients. By no means all of them, however, were suffering from dizziness. He did not include tests for positional nystagmus amongst his investigations. In an address to the Royal Society of Medicine, Cawthorne (1946) described a series of studies on 58 head-injured patients; he compared their symptoms with those of a group in whom labyrinthectomy had been performed for Ménière's disease. Only two of the 58 patients studied had normal caloric responses and, on the basis of this and the similarity of symptoms in the two groups, he concluded that persistent vertigo after concussion was likely to be due to vestibular end-organ damage. By now the work of Dix and Hallpike (1952) was becoming increasingly recognized, and two UK studies of positional nystagmus in post-traumatic vertigo were published within two years of each other: those of Gordon (1954) and Harrison (1956). In the first of these, Gordon described briefly the history of positional nystagmus and referred to the description of the syndrome of benign positional vertigo by Dix and Hallpike (1952). Likening the symptoms of this syndrome to that of many patients with post-traumatic dizziness, Gordon described five patients with dizziness after head injury, all of whom had positional nystagmus of the so-called peripheral type. In a larger study, Harrison (1956) described his findings in a series of 108 unselected patients with head injury, of whom 17 (15 per cent) showed positional nystagmus of the benign paroxysmal type. Fifteen of these 17 cases had a complaint of rotational dizziness, whereas only three of the 91 without nystagmus had such a complaint. Harrison emphasized the unreliability of caloric testing in this syndrome.

By this stage an extensive literature on positional nystagmus had accumulated. Early on, Nylén (1950) had suggested a classification, but it was criticized by Aschan, Bergstedt and Stahle (1956) and Fernandés and Lindsay (1960) because it disregarded the duration of the nystagmus. Since then, largely on the basis of the work of Dix and Hallpike (1952) and Aschan, Bergstedt and Stahle (1956), two distinct types of positional nystagmus have been defined:

Type one — nystagmus induced by sudden change in position of the head and persisting for as long as the position is maintained. It is not accompanied by constant vertigo.

Type two — nystagmus induced in the same way that is of short duration, but associated with pronounced vertigo. In this type, which is thought to be peripheral in origin, there tends to be a latent period between the positional change and the onset of nystagmus. Furthermore the response fatigues with repeated attempts to elicit it. It is Type two, peripheral labyrinthine positional nystagmus, which most commonly occurs in patients with post-traumatic dizziness.

In more recent discussion on the subject of positional vertigo, Harrison and Ozsahinoglu (1972) refer to a third type of positional nystagmus. It consists of a mixture of Type one and Type two characteristics and is accompanied by severe vertigo. In the study these authors described, head injury was responsible for 17 per cent of those cases with Type one, 24 per cent of those with Type two and 17 per cent of those with Type three nystagmus.

Clearly the evidence so far would suggest that post-traumatic vertigo is commonly a result of organic vestibular disturbance. The problem remains of whether the damage to vestibular pathways from head injury is placed centrally in the brain stem or peripherally in the labyrinth. Amongst the early proponents of the central theory were Proctor, Gurdjian and Webster (1956), but in their paper they did not advance a great deal of evidence in support of their theory. A peripheral cause for post-traumatic vertigo was supported by Barber (1964). He reached his conclusions largely on the basis of the type of positional nystagmus that he detected clinically. He also took particular care in his analysis of clinical symptoms and sought to make a distinction between true spinning sensations and less marked feelings of faintness, swaying, swimming, etc., which may nevertheless bespeak organic vestibular imbalance. He made the important clinical point that 'regarding positional vertigo and nystagmus, the keyword is *bed*. Characteristically, he explains, 'this group of patients relate objective rotational spinning of their surroundings when they first lie supine in bed at night, or upon arising from bed in the morning, or on rolling over on to one or the other side; they may even be awakened from sleep by vertigo, realising afterward that they have turned to one side while asleep.' In his series, Barber (1964) included 165 patients with dizziness after head injury, and 25 per cent of them had positional nystagmus. As noted above (Harrison and Ozsahinoglu, 1972) head injuries may produce a variety of different types of positional nystagmus. The correlation between the site of the lesion and the type of nystagmus is probably less clear than was thought at one time. Most workers would now take the view that the clinical characteristics of positional nystagmus cannot in all cases be relied upon to distinguish between central and peripheral vestibular lesions.

Recently it has been found that the brainstem auditory-evoked potentials may be abnormal in some patients with dizziness after a minor head injury (Rowe and Carlson, 1980). Whilst this would tend to support a central cause for the dizziness, further studies using this technique are required.

Pathological Studies

Let us now consider some of the pathological evidence for a correlation between vestibular damage and a history of post-traumatic dizziness, taking into account the information available on both central and peripheral lesions. It is well known that head trauma, even in absence of skull fracture or gross intracranial pathology, may damage the central nervous system at the cellular level. One of the earliest relevant descriptions was by Windle, Groat and Fox (1944), who showed that in experimental animals changes in the vestibular nuclei commonly occurred after head injury. In man, pathological changes in the brain stem of patients dying from head injury are common (Tomlinson, 1970; Crompton, 1971). Of Crompton's 106 patients studied pathologically, 13 showed evidence of neuronal degeneration in vestibular nuclei; he thought that the changes probably resulted from the shearing force of the primary impact. The demonstration of such findings in cases of severe head injury cannot, of course, be regarded as evidence for a central vestibular cause of post-traumatic dizziness in patients who survive their head injuries. We are not aware of any instance where a patient with post-traumatic vertigo as a result of minor head injury has subsequently been shown to have a central vestibular abnormality at later post mortem.

The temporal bone is frequently involved in head trauma, and the ear is said to be the most frequently damaged sensory organ of the body (Hough and Stewart, 1968). Schuknecht and Davison (1956) showed that cats subjected to experimental head trauma developed tears in the membranous walls of the utricle and saccule, and there was a decrease in the hair cell population of the saccular macula. They thought that damage to the utricle was probably responsible both for benign positional vertigo and for post-traumatic vertigo. Futhermore, they speculated on the possible role of the otoconia in the production of positional vertigo and nystagmus: they thought that a blow to the head could cause disruption of the otolithic membrane and detachment of otoconia. The latter when floating freely might settle in the most dependent part of the labyrinth, namely the posterior semicircular canal. Certain changes in head position could cause the otoconia to act upon the cupola of this canal and thus produce the symptoms and the nystagmus (Schuknecht, 1969). Attempts to test this theory have been hampered by the fact that otoconia cannot be identified clearly in decalcified histological preparations.

In recent years there has been extensive study of temporal bone fractures both from the clinical, pathological and radiological points of view (Hough, 1970; Mathog, 1971; Potter, 1972; Laszlo, 1973). Not all patients with post-traumatic dizziness have detectable fractures, but it is well known that these may be very difficult to demonstrate radiologically. What can be said is that when a fracture is present, post-traumatic dizziness is common. In Barber's (1964) series of 47 longitudinal temporal bone fractures, positional nystagmus was observed in 47 per cent, in contrast to its occurrence in 21 per cent of a group of 77 patients with injuries of comparable severity but without fracture.

Further evidence to support a peripheral labyrinthine cause for post-traumatic vertigo was produced by Steffen (1965) in a report on three cases. In two of them there had been persisting positional dizziness, in one case for nine years and in the other for 14 months, and in both of them section of the appropriate vestibular nerve was said to relieve their symptoms.

Electronystagmography

The introduction of the technique of electronystagmography has revolutionized the assessment of nystagmus, as it is now possible to produce an objective record of the nystagmus which can be repeated as often as necessary. Apart from its objectivity, the other obvious advantage of electronystagmography is that it allows recording with the eyes closed. There is evidence to suggest that it may be possible to differentiate central from peripheral vestibular nystagmus on the basis of the changing characteristics when eyes are open or closed (see Table 10.1). The early literature on the recording of eye movements is summarized by Aschan, Bergstedt and Stahle (1956) and by Jongkees and Philipszoon (1963); more recent reviews of the technique provide further testimony as to its usefulness (Rubin, 1969; Cox and Spongberg, 1972; Eviator, 1972). Toglia has made a number of further contributions to the subject (Toglia, 1969; Toglia,

Rosenberg and Ronis, 1970; Toglia, 1972). Using electronystagmography, he studied large numbers of patients suffering from post-traumatic dizziness, and has found abnormalities in as many as two-thirds. He has discussed the role of the electronystagmogram in the assessment of these patients, and he makes the point that the presence of positional nystagmus, as seen clinically or as demonstrated electrically, provides strong evidence that the patient's symptoms are, in part at least, organic in nature.

Valuable though it is, electronystagmography in patients with post-traumatic dizziness does not allow a certain differentiation between a central or peripheral labyrinthine cause. Current evidence would suggest that both may occur; but, as we shall see later, our own experience suggests that a peripheral disturbance is the most common cause of post-traumatic vertigo.

Table 10.1. Effects of eye closure and darkness upon spontaneous nystagmus resulting from lesions at different levels of the CNS.

Lesion	Darkness	Eye closure
Labyrynthine or peripheral to vestibular nuclei	Nystagmus enhanced if present or made manifest if not	Nystagmus enhanced if present or made manifest if not
At or about the level of the vestibular nuclei	Nystagmus enhanced in amplitude but decreased in respect of slow component velocity	Nystagmus abolished
Above the level of the vestibular nuclei	Nystagmus abolished	Nystagmus abolished

From Hood, J. D. (1968) Electronystagmography. *Journal of Laryngology and Otology,* **82,** 67-183, with kind permission of the author and publisher.

Conclusions

During the past 100 years it has become increasingly recognized that dizziness and vertigo may commonly occur as a result of head injury. Current evidence suggests that in the majority of patients these symptoms are caused by a disturbance of the vestibular apparatus, either in the brain stem or in the labyrinth (evidence in favour of the latter being more convincing). The roles of psychological factors, vasomotor instability and the so-called cervical syndrome in the production of post-traumatic dizziness and vertigo are uncertain.

THE NEWCASTLE SERIES

The symptom of dizziness in the Newcastle patients was assessed in the same way as headache. Patients were interviewed in a particular and exact manner during hospitalization, on discharge and at follow-up visits. They were initially asked if they had any symptoms, and if at this stage dizziness was offered 'spontaneously' it was recorded as such. A more specific enquiry was made if a symptom was not volunteered at the first time of asking, and if one was forthcoming on the second round it was recorded as 'present with prompting'. Finally, the patients were asked about a variety of symptoms, as noted in the symptom inventory (see Table 9.3), and invited to comment on each in turn. If dizziness was admitted in this circumstance it was scored as 'present on direct questioning'.

Early Post-traumatic Dizziness

'Early dizziness' was defined as that occurring during hospitalization or on discharge. Seventy-two of the patients complained of dizziness during hospitalization (Table 10.2), and on discharge the same 72 patients were still complaining of it.

Table 10.2. Numbers of patients with dizziness (Newcastle series).

	Dizziness		Total patients
	No.	(%)	
During hospitalization	72	19	372
On discharge	72	19	372
At 6 months	74	22	338
At 1 year	45	14	323
At 2 years	54	18	300

Dizziness was described in a variety of ways, but we have as far as possible divided the patients into just two groups: those with true rotational vertigo and those with other forms of dizziness (Table 10.3). On discharge, 80 per cent of the patients with dizziness had true vertigo. Almost half of those who offered dizziness as a symptom at the time of discharge did so spontaneously; about a quarter responded only to a direct question (Table 10.4).

Table 10.3. Types of dizziness (Newcastle series).

	Vertigo		Other dizziness		Total with dizziness
	No.	(%)	No.	(%)	
On discharge	58	80	14	20	72
At 6 months	37	50	37	50	74
At 1 year	22	49	23	51	45
At 2 years	16	29	38	71	54

We have looked at a variety of factors in relation to early post-traumatic dizziness. The age and sex distribution of affected patients showed a slight variation from that of the whole population studied (Tables 10.5 and 10.6). There was a higher-than-expected proportion of females among those with dizziness at the time of discharge, and the mean age of those with dizziness was higher than that of non-sufferers, particularly in the two-year follow-up group. There was no obvious association between the development of dizziness and the type of accident sustained; nor was there any particular importance attaching to the exact site of the injury. Social class did not seem to be a factor of any significance in relation to the development of dizziness. Neither did severity of head injury correlate with the occurrence of early post-traumatic

Table 10.4. Dizziness on discharge (Newcastle series).

	No. of cases	(%)
'Spontaneous'	34	48
'Prompting'	19	26
'Direct questioning'	19	26
Total	72	100

dizziness. Quite a high proportion of those with dizziness had had short periods of post-traumatic amnesia of less than an hour (Table 10.7). Again there is no evidence that dizziness was more common in those with skull fracture (Table 10.8).

We have attempted to relate the occurrence of early post-traumatic dizziness to other symptoms noted on the symptom inventory. It transpires that impairment of concentration, anxiety and, in particular, headache were all encountered more frequently by those with dizziness than by those without it (Table 10.9). The inter-relationship of these symptoms will be discussed later when we come to consider the postconcussional syndrome.

Table 10.5. Mean age (years) of patients with dizziness (Newcastle series).

	Male	Female	All patients
Discharge	38.90 (37.67)*	47.40 (42.07)*	42.44 (38.94)*
6 months	43.23 (37.05)*	48.22 (49.24)*	45.05 (40.69)*
1 year	45.67 (36.46)*	44.00 (47.88)*	45.56 (39.89)*
2 years	53.88 (35.68)*	52.60 (48.22)*	53.41 (39.41)*

*Figures in brackets indicate mean ages (years) of whole study population.

During the early part of the study it soon became apparent that a significant percentage of patients with early post-traumatic dizziness had positional nystagmus and, from Case 76 onwards, all patients were specifically tested for it whether or not they complained of dizziness. In the event, positional nystagmus was not seen in any patient who did not have a complaint of dizziness. Table 10.10 details the incidence of positional nystagmus in those with dizziness on discharge from hospital. Just over a quarter were found to have positional nystagmus and the proportion was highest in those patients with true vertigo, although it was occasionally found in patients with other types of dizziness.

To summarize thus far, no particular characteristic seems to identify those patients most likely to have dizziness in the early stages after head injury. Early post-

Table 10.6. Male/female distribution of dizziness on discharge.

	Present		Absent		Total	
	No.	(%)	No.	(%)	No.	(%)
Male	42	58	222	74	264	71
Female	30	42	78	26	108	29
Total	72	100	300	100	372	100

Table 10.7. Dizziness at discharge related to period of post-traumatic amnesia (Newcastle series).

Period of post-traumatic amnesia	Dizziness				Total	
	Present		Absent			
	No.	(%)	No.	(%)	No.	(%)
Nil	7		31		38	
< 1 minute	7		14		21	
1—5 minutes	10	48 (67)	29	137 (53)	39	185 (56)
6—15 minutes	7		10		17	
16—60 minutes	17		53		70	
1—6 hours	4		40		44	
7—12 hours	4		8		12	
13—24 hours	5	24 (33)	13	121 (47)	18	145 (44)
1—7 days	5		32		37	
> 7 days	6		28		34	
Total	72	*(100)*	258	*(100)*	330	*(100)*
Unknown	0		42		42	
All patients	72		300		372	

traumatic dizziness appears to be more common in women, but does not relate to the severity of the injury, its site on the head, or the presence or absence of skull fracture. Patients with early post-traumatic dizziness often have other symptoms, such as headache; they complain of dizziness spontaneously and over a quarter of them show evidence of positional nystagmus.

Table 10.8. Dizziness on discharge related to skull fracture (Newcastle series).

Skull fracture	Dizziness				Total	
	Present		Absent			
	No.	(%)	No.	(%)	No.	(%)
Present	18	27	70	24	88	24
Absent	49	73	225	76	274	76
No X-ray	5		5		10	
Total	72	*100*	300	*100*	372	*100*

Persisting Post-traumatic Dizziness

The proportion of patients with post-traumatic dizziness seems to remain remarkably stable at the various periods of follow-up (Table 10.2). As with headache, this might be because a patient with a particular symptom was more likely to attend the clinic regularly but, as we have noted previously, our follow-up procedure attempted to circumvent this possibility.

The sex distribution of patients with dizziness after discharge from hospital did not differ from that of those without it. The mean age of patients with dizziness did appear to differ from the overall mean, those with dizziness being older (Table 10.5). The males with persisting post-traumatic dizziness two years after discharge had a mean age that was quite strikingly different from that of the total population (Table 10.5).

Table 10.9. Dizziness on discharge related to other symptoms (Newcastle series).

Symptoms	Patients with dizziness		All patients	
	No.	(%)	No.	(%)
Total	72		372	
Depression	7	10	31	8
Impaired concentration	10	14	14	4
Anxiety	11	15	29	8
Headache	55	76	135	36

As in the case of early post-traumatic dizziness, we have attempted to correlate persisting dizziness with a number of other variables. It does not appear to relate to social class, to site of injury or to type of injury. Although there was no increased incidence of skull fracture in patients with early dizziness, this was not true of those with late dizziness; at the various follow-up visits there appeared to be an above-average incidence of skull fracture in those with dizziness (Table 10.11). There was no significant correlation between the duration of post-traumatic amnesia and the occurrence of dizziness, at any stage (Table 10.12); in other words, the figures do not suggest a positive correlation between the incidence of post-traumatic dizziness and the severity of injury.

Table 10.10. Dizziness on discharge and positional nystagmus (PN) (Newcastle series).

	PN		Total
	No.	(%)	
Vertigo	19	33	58
Other dizziness	2	14	14
Total with dizziness	*21*	*29*	*72*

With the passage of time there was a gradual fall-off in the numbers of patients complaining spontaneously of dizziness (Table 10.13). At the two-year follow-up, two-thirds of those complaining of dizziness did so only in response to direct questioning, while only about 10 per cent complained of the symptom spontaneously.

The relationship between dizziness and symptoms of depression, impairment of concentration, anxiety and headache have been examined with respect to the six-month, one-year and two-year follow-ups (Tables 10.14, 10.15 and 10.16). With the exception of anxiety, the symptoms mentioned are all more common in patients with dizziness than in the head injury population as a whole.

The incidence of positional nystagmus amongst the patients with dizziness has been examined at time of discharge and at each follow-up period (Table 10.17). Table 10.17 includes the combined figures for all patients with dizziness and also gives a break-down into patients with vertigo and those with other forms of dizziness. The number of patients with persisting dizziness remains high, even at two years, although there is a substantial decline in the incidence of positional nystagmus during that period. The relationship between positional nystagmus at time of discharge and the

Table 10.11. Dizziness on discharge and at follow-up in relation to skull fracture (Newcastle series).

Skull fracture	All patients on discharge		Dizziness							
			On discharge		At 6 months		At 1 year		At 2 years	
	No.	(%)	No.	(%)	No.	(%)	No.	(%)	No.	(%)
Present	88	24	18	27	23	32	21	47	20	37
Absent	274	76	49	73	49	73	24	53	34	63
No X-ray	10		5		2		0		0	
Total	*372*		*72*		*74*		*45*		*54*	

Table 10.12. Dizziness on discharge and at follow-up related to post-traumatic amnesia (Newcastle series).

	Dizziness								Total patients	
	Discharge		6 months		1 year		2 years			
	No.	(%)	No.	(%)	No.	(%)	No.	(%)	No.	(%)
PTA: <1 hour	48	67	46	62	30	67	35	65	185	56
>1 hour	24	33	28	38	15	33	19	35	145	44
Total with dizziness	*72*		*74*		*45*		*54*			
Total patients	372		338		323		300		372	

Table 10.13. Dizziness on discharge and at follow-up (Newcastle series).

	Discharge		6 months		1 year		2 years	
	No.	(%)	No.	(%)	No.	(%)	No.	(%)
'Spontaneous'	34	48	26	35	6	13	6	11
'Prompting'	19	26	20	27	16	36	12	22
'Direct questioning'	19	26	28	38	23	51	36	67
Total	*72*		*74*		*45*		*54*	

Table 10.14. Dizziness and other symptoms at 6 months (Newcastle series).

Symptoms	Patients with dizziness		All patients	
	No.	(%)	No.	(%)
Total	74		338	
Depression	20	27	60	18
Impaired concentration	11	15	21	6
Anxiety	12	16	40	12
Headache	44	59	91	27

Table 10.15. Dizziness and other symptoms at 1 year (Newcastle series).

Symptoms	Patients with dizziness		All patients	
	No.	(%)	No.	(%)
Total	45		323	
Depression	11	24	58	18
Impaired concentration	14	31	32	10
Anxiety	5	11	45	14
Headache	16	36	58	18

persistence of dizziness at the various follow-up periods is shown in Table 10.18. Twenty-one of the patients who were dizzy on discharge had positional nystagmus at the time. Of the 74 patients who were dizzy at six months, 14 (19 per cent) had had nystagmus at the time of discharge. At the one-year follow-up there were still 45 patients with dizziness, and 8 of them had had positional nystagmus on discharge. At the two-year follow-up 54 patients were recorded as having dizziness and 8 of them had had early positional nystagmus.

Table 10.16. Dizziness and other symptoms at 2 years (Newcastle series).

Symptoms	Patients with dizziness		All patients	
	No.	(%)	No.	(%)
Total	54		300	
Depression	19	35	56	19
Impaired concentration	17	31	33	11
Anxiety	8	15	48	16
Headache	27	50	72	24

In a previous chapter we have commented on the numbers of patients who were pursuing claims for compensation at the various follow-up intervals. At six months 26 per cent were doing so. At one and two years the figures were 31 per cent and 33 per cent respectively. The figures were higher when we looked separately at patients with dizziness. At six months 39 per cent were pursuing claims, at one year 51 per cent and at two years 50 per cent.

The figures we have been examining suggest that there are slight differences between patients with early post-traumatic dizziness and patients with late persistence of the symptom. As was the case with headache, the prospective design of the study

Table 10.17. Dizziness and positional nystagmus on discharge and at follow-up (Newcastle series).

	Vertigo			Other dizziness			Total with dizziness		
	Total	Positional nystagmus No.	(%)	Total	Positional nystagmus No.	(%)	Total	Positional nystagmus No.	(%)
Discharge	58	19	33	14	2	14	72	21	29
6 months	37	12	32	37	5	14	74	17	23
1 year	22	3	14	23	2	9	45	5	11
2 years	16	2	13	38	2	5	54	4	7

Table 10.18. Nystagmus on discharge related to dizziness during follow-up (Newcastle series).

	Dizziness on discharge	Dizziness at 6 months	Dizziness at 1 year	Dizziness at 2 years
Total with dizziness	72	74	45	54
Nystagmus on discharge	21	14	8	8
Percentage	29	19	18	15

permitted a longitudinal view of patients and symptoms and provided an opportunity to examine the natural history of post-traumatic dizziness in the same way that we examined post-traumatic headache. In Tables 10.19, 10.20 and 10.21 we relate dizziness on discharge from hospital to dizziness at six months, one year and two years. From Table 10.19 it can be seen that, of the 72 patients who had dizziness on discharge, 33 still had persisting dizziness at six months, 31 patients had improved and 8 had been lost to follow-up. A total of 74 patients had dizziness at the six-month follow-up; 33 had had it since the time of discharge but no less than 41 patients had acquired the symptom in the interval between discharge and the six-month follow-up. By the end of

Table 10.19. Patients with dizziness on discharge and at 6 months (Newcastle series).

	Dizziness at 6 months		Lost to follow-up	Total
	Present	Absent		
Dizziness on discharge:				
Present	33	31	8	72
Absent	41	233	26	300
Total	74	264	34	372

two years, just over half the patients with dizziness on discharge had improved, whilst 32 patients not complaining of dizziness on discharge had since acquired it (Table 10.21). Thus the figures show quite clearly that the patients with persistent dizziness at six months, one year and two years after discharge comprise two groups: those in whom it was genuinely persistent throughout follow-up, and those who developed it during the course of follow-up. As in the case of headache, we have used the terms 'persisting' and 'late acquired' to identify the two groups. They were analysed separately in relation to positional nystagmus, depression and involvement in compensation in each follow-up period (Tables 10.22, 10.23 and 10.24). It is interesting to note that whilst the 'persisting' and 'late-acquired' groups do not differ

Table 10.20. Patients with dizziness on discharge and at 1 year (Newcastle series).

	Dizziness at 1 year		Lost to follow-up	Total
	Present	Absent		
Dizziness on discharge:				
Present	25	38	9	72
Absent	20	240	40	300
Total	45	278	49	372

Table 10.21. Patients with dizziness on discharge and at 2 years (Newcastle series).

	Dizziness at 2 years		Lost to follow-up	Total
	Present	Absent		
Dizziness on discharge:				
Present	22	38	12	72
Absent	32	208	60	300
Total	*54*	*246*	*72*	*372*

Table 10.22. Factors related to dizziness at 6 months (Newcastle series).

	Total	Compensation		Depression		Positional nystagmus	
		No.	(%)	No.	(%)	No.	(%)
Dizziness:							
Persisting	33	8	24	4	12	15	45
Late-acquired	41	21	51	16	39	2	5
Total	74	29	39	20	27	17	23
All patients	338	88	26	60	18	17	5

Table 10.23. Factors related to dizziness at 1 year (Newcastle series).

	Total	Compensation		Depression		Positional nystagmus	
		No.	(%)	No.	(%)	No.	(%)
Dizziness:							
Persisting	25	8	32	4	16	5	20
Late-acquired	20	15	75	7	35	0	
Total	45	23	51	11	24	5	11
All patients	323	100	31	58	18	5	2

Table 10.24. Factors related to dizziness at 2 years (Newcastle series).

	Total	Compensation		Depression		Positional nystagmus	
		No.	(%)	No.	(%)	No.	(%)
Dizziness:							
Persisting	22	7	32	5	23	4	18
Late-acquired	32	20	63	14	44	0	
Total	54	27	50	19	35	4	7
All patients	300	100	33	56	19	4	1

in age, sex, presence or absence of skull fracture, and severity of injury (as measured by length of post-traumatic amnesia) they do show a striking difference in the incidence of positional nystagmus and depression and in the numbers of patients involved in compensation claims.

Depression

In Chapter Eight it was stated that depression had been diagnosed in about one-fifth of all patients seen at follow-up visits. In the group of patients with post-traumatic dizziness the proportion is slightly higher. Perhaps the most significant observation is that whilst slightly less than a quarter of those with 'persisting' dizziness developed depression, between one-third and a half of patients with 'late acquired' dizziness did so. This point will be discussed again when we come to consider the postconcussional syndrome.

Compensation

It is of some interest to look at the relationship between the prevalence of dizziness at the various follow-up times and the pursuit of compensation claims. The picture that emerges is similar to that seen in the case of post-traumatic headache, considered in the last chapter. In Table 10.25, patients are divided into two groups according to the presence or absence of dizziness. The percentages making claims at the time of each follow-up examination are recorded for both groups. It can be seen that there were

Table 10.25. Compensation claims in patients with and without dizziness (Newcastle series).

	At 6 months (%)	At 1 year (%)	At 2 years (%)
Dizziness present	39	51	50
Dizziness absent	22	28	31

considerably more claims in the dizziness group than in the 'no dizziness' group. In Table 10.26, the dizziness group has been subdivided into 'persisting' and 'late acquired' categories, that is, those whose dizziness continued from the time that they were in hospital, and those who had developed dizziness during one of the follow-up periods. The table shows that there were more claimants amongst those in the 'late acquired' group. This would seem to support the clinical impression that a substantial part, though not all, of the dizziness complained of by those pursuing compensation claims is of a functional nature. Our own belief is that the majority of those who have true organic dizziness will have a characteristic history of positional provocation and will have demonstrable nystagmus on tipping.

Table 10.26. Compensation claims in patients with 'persisting' and 'late acquired' dizziness (Newcastle series).

	At 6 months (%)	At 1 year (%)	At 2 years (%)
Persisting dizziness	24	32	32
Late acquired dizziness	51	75	63
All patients with dizziness	39	51	50

Positional Nystagmus

At an early stage in the study it became apparent that positional nystagmus was common in patients with early post-traumatic dizziness. Positional nystagmus is undoubtedly a very useful clinical sign for, when present, it clearly indicates an organic basis for the symptom of dizziness. Nevertheless the sign is not infallible and its absence cannot be regarded as excluding absolutely an organic cause. One point does emerge quite clearly from our own figures. Patients with what we have called 'late-acquired' post-traumatic dizziness are very unlikely to show positional nystagmus.

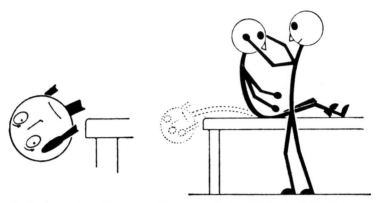

Figure 10.1. Cawthorne positional test. From Cawthorne, T., Dix, M. R., Hallpike, C. S. and Hood, J. D. (1956) The investigation of vestibular function. *Brit. Med. Bull.* 12: 131-142, with kind permission of the author and the *British Medical Bulletin*.

The clinical test for positional nystagmus is easy to perform and to observe (Figure 10.1), but in order to examine more closely the detailed features of the nystagmus we have used a crude recording system. Two channels of a 12-channel EEG machine were used; the electrode positions are illustrated in Figure 10.2. Patients were seated in a dental

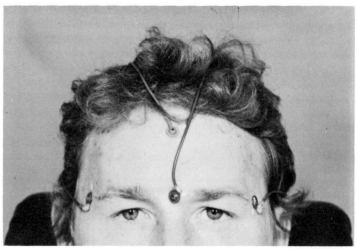

Figure 10.2. Electrode positions.

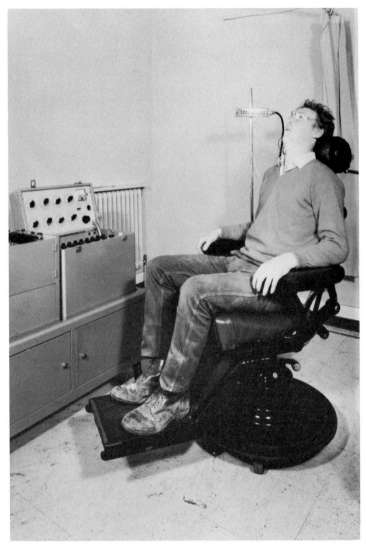

Figure 10.3. Seating arrangement for recording.

chair (Figure 10.3) and recordings were made while tipping to the horizontal position with the head turned to one side (Figure 10.4).

The technique of electronystagmography depends upon the differential polarity of the eye — the front of the eye is positively charged in relation to the back. With appropriate electrode placements, horizontal movements of the eye may be recorded by deflections on either a d.c. or an a.c. recorder (Figure 10.5). We used this technique to examine all 21 patients who had clinical evidence of positional nystagmus at the time of their discharge from hospital, and in all of them the nystagmus could be recorded electrically. We also used the technique to examine a further 30 patients in the study who did not have positional nystagmus but who complained of dizziness at the time

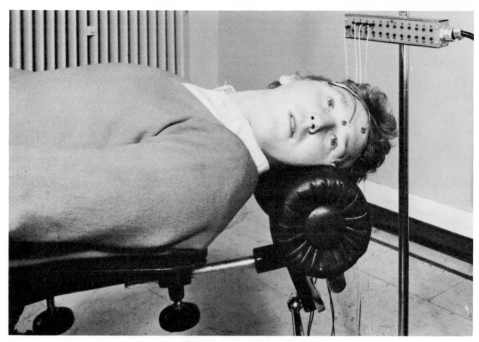

Figure 10.4. Position of head during tipping.

they left hospital. In only two of them could positional nystagmus be recorded on the ENG. Although we would not regard electronystagmography as an essential routine diagnostic method, we have found it useful for the study of the natural history of positional nystagmus in patients with post-traumatic dizziness, perhaps providing some pointers to its possible pathological basis.

Some idea of the relationship between clinically observed and electrically recorded positional nystagmus can be gained from Table 10.27, which gives details of the findings in the 72 patients who complained of dizziness on discharge from hospital. Of

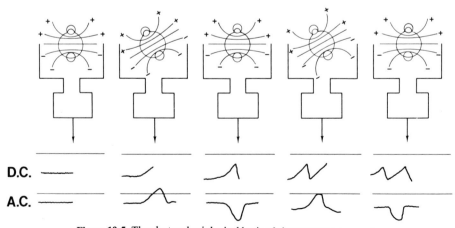

Figure 10.5. The electrophysiological basis of electronystagmography.

Table 10.27. Dizziness on discharge, the incidence of positional nystagmus (PN) and ENG abnormalities (Newcastle series).

Dizziness on discharge

	72		
PN not seen	51	21	PN seen
ENG tested	30	21	ENG tested
PN recorded	2	21	PN recorded
Total positive		23	

these 72 patients, 21 had clinically detectable nystagmus and, as indicated above, it could invariably be demonstrated electrically. Of the 51 patients who had dizziness on discharge from hospital but who did not have clinically demonstrable positional nystagmus, 30 were investigated by means of the ENG. In only two of them was nystagmus recorded, so it would appear that in early post-traumatic dizziness our ENG system is only slightly more sensitive than is clinical examination for detecting positional nystagmus.

Six normal volunteers were submitted to electronystagmography and in no instance was positional nystagmus recorded. It has been claimed that some normal people do show the phenomenon but this has not been our experience. Our own studies suggest that the rather crude technique that we have employed is not sensitive enough to detect anything less than gross positional nystagmus. Despite this, the technique was of some value in the detection of positional nystagmus at the follow-up visits. Table 10.28 gives details of the numbers of patients with dizziness at the various follow-up periods and indicates those in whom positional nystagmus was demonstrated clinically and electrically. All patients previously shown clinically to have positional nystagmus were tested with the ENG at each follow-up visit; it can be seen from the table that at the two-year follow-up the ENG was positive in nine patients, although the nystagmus could be seen clinically in only four of them. We believe that the explanation for this is not that the ENG is a more sensitive test but rather that it allows the recording of the nystagmus when the patients have their eyes closed. In our experience, positional nystagmus after head injury is often more readily recorded with the eyes closed than with them open. Patients were tested first with eyes open and subsequently with them closed. Of the 23 patients in whom nystagmus was recorded on ENG at the time of discharge from hospital, five had nystagmus that could be recorded only with eyes open, 16 had nystagmus that was enhanced with eye closure and two had nystagmus that could be recorded only with the eyes closed. In these two it obviously could not be demonstrated clinically. At the six-month follow-up, seven patients had

Table 10.28. Dizziness, positional nystagmus and electronystagmography (Newcastle series).

	Dizziness	Positional nystagmus seen	ENG tested	ENG positive
Discharge	72	21	51	23
6 months	74	17	20	19
1 year	45	5	15	10
2 years	54	4	12	9

nystagmus recorded only with eyes open, ten had nystagmus that was enhanced by eye closure and in two it could be recorded only with eyes closed. At one year, five patients had nystagmus enhanced by eye closure and five had nystagmus that was detectable only with eyes closed. Finally, at the two-year follow-up, four patients had nystagmus enhanced by eye closure and the remaining five with a positive recording all had to have their eyes closed to obtain it. In other words, it was our experience that nystagmus in the majority of patients was enhanced with eye closure, which would argue strongly in favour of a peripheral labyrinthine disturbance as a cause for the post-traumatic dizziness.

Some typical features of the post-traumatic positional vertigo syndrome were encountered in Case 194, a 62-year-old female who suffered a relatively mild head injury when she was knocked over by a bus. Her period of post-traumatic amnesia was estimated at five minutes, yet from the time of the accident she complained of quite severe dizziness brought on by any head movement and particularly by looking upwards at the ceiling and by lying down or turning over in bed. When she was tipped with her head to the right, marked rotary nystagmus was seen easily after a few seconds' delay. Repetition of the test showed that the nystagmus readily fatigued. ENGs were recorded (Figures 10.6 to 10.12).

Figure 10.6 shows the eye movements on looking ahead, to the left, to the right and vertically; no spontaneous nystagmus is visible. This recording was made three weeks after the injury. Figure 10.7 is the recording of a series of runs after tipping with the eyes open, and nystagmus is demonstrated after a few seconds' delay.

The patient still complained of positional dizziness approximately two months after these recordings were made, but the ENG with eyes open showed only occasional beats of nystagmus (Fig 10.8). When the test was repeated with eyes closed (Fig 10.9), nystagmus was clearly seen and it could still be recorded on a second run. A further three months on, nystagmus could not be recorded with eyes open, but with eyes closed it was still clearly recordable (Fig 10.10). Seven months after the accident the patient still complained of dizziness, but positional nystagmus could not be seen, nor could it be recorded electrically with the eyes open (Fig 10.11). With the eyes closed, however, nystagmus could still be recorded (Fig 10.12). Even at the two-year follow-up this patient still had positional nystagmus which could be recorded with the eyes closed, although it could not be seen clinically or recorded with eyes open.

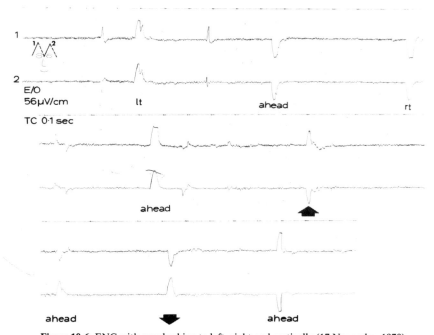

Figure 10.6. ENG with eyes looking to left, right and vertically (17 November 1970).

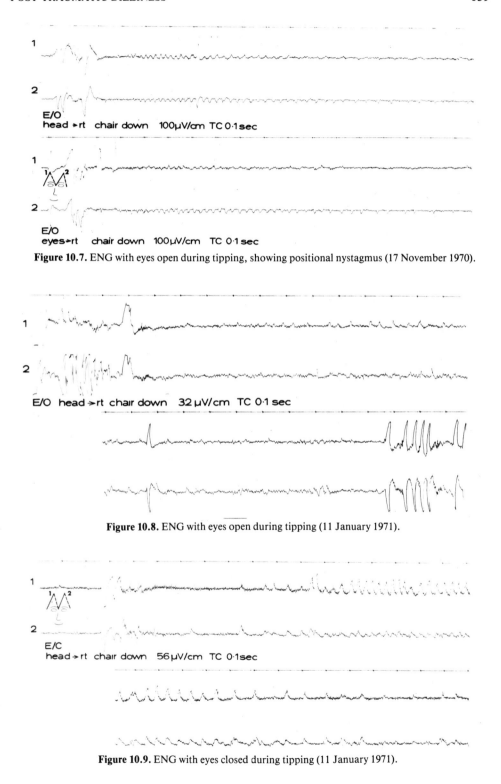

Figure 10.7. ENG with eyes open during tipping, showing positional nystagmus (17 November 1970).

Figure 10.8. ENG with eyes open during tipping (11 January 1971).

Figure 10.9. ENG with eyes closed during tipping (11 January 1971).

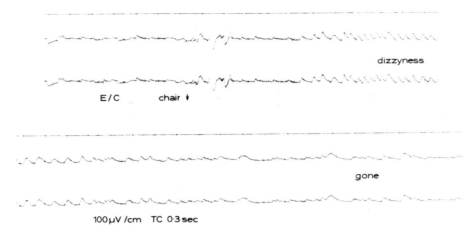

dizzyness

E/C   chair ↓

gone

100μV/cm   TC 0·3 sec

Figure 10.10. ENG with eyes closed during tipping (24 April 1971).

On the basis of the clinical and electrical characteristics that we have observed, it is our belief that a significant proportion of patients with positional nystagmus and dizziness after head injury have damage in their labyrinths. It seems probable that such labyrinthine disturbances are the commonest cause of early post-traumatic dizziness, but we were unable to demonstrate their existence in all our patients.

What other possible explanations for post-traumatic dizziness might there be? We considered the possible role of so-called 'vasomotor instability'; all 72 patients with dizziness on discharge from hospital were examined carefully for the presence of orthostatic hypotension. In none could a significant fall in blood pressure be demonstrated. In all of them, we also carried out a relatively crude examination of the

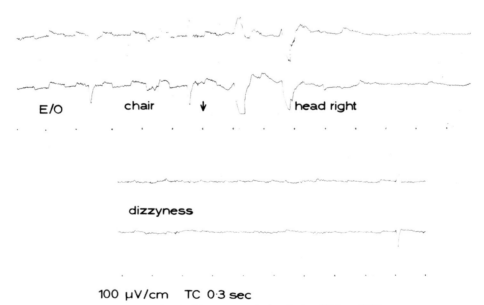

E/O   chair   ↓   head right

dizzyness

100 μV/cm   TC 0·3 sec

Figure 10.11. ENG with eyes open during tipping (24 June 1971).

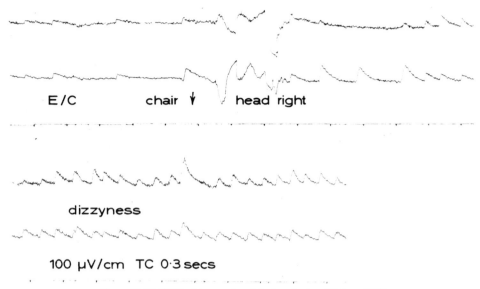

E/C   chair ↓   head right

dizzyness

100 µV/cm   TC 0·3 secs

Figure 10.12. ENG with eyes closed during tipping (24 June 1971).

baroreceptor response to a Valsalva manoeuvre, using the De Bono device (De Bono, 1963). It consists of a small needle attached to a narrow gauge plastic tube with a sealed end. The needle is inserted into the brachial artery and blood fills the plastic tube, except for a small gap at the end, which contains compressed air. The character of the arterial pulsation and the changes in blood pressure can readily be observed during the performance of the Valsalva manoeuvre and the characteristic arterial blood pressure overshoot can readily be observed. In our 72 patients with dizziness the response was perfectly normal, thus providing further evidence that there was no disturbance of their vasomotor reflexes.

Persisting and Late Acquired Post-traumatic Dizziness

As was noted in the case of headache, we see our patients with post-discharge dizziness dividing into two groups. Those with 'persisting' dizziness appear in the main to have an organic basis for their symptoms. Positional nystagmus recorded clinically or electrically occurred in this group and was seen in many instances through to the two-year follow-up visit. In patients who acquire post-traumatic dizziness two factors of importance are encountered: depression and legal proceedings. Our figures suggest that depression may play an important role in the causation of post-traumatic dizziness in about a third of the patients. In the next chapter we shall consider the association between the late development of dizziness and headache, which are so often encountered together.

SUMMARY OF CONCLUSIONS

On the basis of the Newcastle study we have concluded that a significant proportion of patients with early post-traumatic dizziness have evidence of peripheral labyrinthine damage. Early post-traumatic dizziness does tend to improve in the early months following injury; approximately half of our patients had recovered by the end of six months, although in some patients dizziness persisted for as long as two years after head injury. In these patients, evidence of labyrinthine damage may still be found sometimes and even after two years electronystagmographic abnormality may still be seen.

We have found that a number of patients develop dizziness after they have been discharged from hospital. In this group it is exceptional to find objective evidence of organic damage. A high proportion of these patients are involved in claims for compensation, and over a third of them show evidence of depression.

REFERENCES

Aschan, G., Bergstedt, M. & Stahle, J. (1956) Nystagmography. *Acta Oto-laryngologica,* Supplement 129.
Bárány, R. (1921) Diagnose von Krankeitserscheinungen in Bereiche des Oto-lithenappareates. *Acta Oto-laryngologica,* **2,** 434-437.
Barber, H. O. (1964) Positional nystagmus, especially after head injury. *Laryngoscope,* **74,** 891-949.
Barré, M. (1926) Sur un syndrome sympathique cervicale posterieur et sa cause frequente; l'arthrite cervicale. *Revue Neurologique,* **6,** 1946-1948.
Bennett, W. (1910) Some milder forms of concussion of the brain. *A System of Medicine.* Allbut, C. & Rolleston, H. D. London: Macmillan.
Biemond, A. & de Jong, J. M. B. V. (1969) On cervical nystagmus and related disorders. *Brain,* **92,** 437-458.
Brunner, H. (1940) Disturbances of the function of the ear after concussion of the brain. *Laryngoscope,* **50,** 921-949.
Caveness, W. F. (1966) Post traumatic sequelae. In *Head Injury* (Ed.) Caveness, W. F. & Walker, A. E. Chapter 17. Philadelphia and Toronto: J. B. Lippincott.
Caveness, W. F. & Nielsen, K. C. (1961) Panel discussion of cerebral concussion and its sequelae. *New York State Medical Journal,* **61,** 1871-1873.
Cawthorne, T. (1946) Vestibular injuries. *Proceedings of The Royal Society of Medicine,* **39,** 270-278.
Compere, W. E. (1968) Electronystagmographic findings in patients with whiplash injuries. *Laryngoscope,* **78,** 1226-1233.
Compere, W. E. (1971) Rheoencephalography in the evaluation of the vertiginous patient. *Laryngoscope,* **81,** 264-272.
Courville, C. (1953) *Commotio cerebri.* Los Angeles: San Lucas Press.
Cox, R. H. & Spongberg, A. K. (1972) Electronystagmography. *Southern Medical Journal,* **65,** 38-40.
Crompton, M. r. (1971) Brain stem lesions due to closed head injury. *Lancet,* **i,** 669-675.
Daremberg, C. V. (1854) *Oevres anatomiques physiologiques et medicales.* Paris: J. B. Bailliere.
Davis, A. G. (1945) Injuries of the cervical spine. *Journal of the American Medical Association,* **127,** 149-156.
De Bono, E. F. (1963) A simple method of intra-arterial pressure measurement. *Lancet,* **i,** 1142-1143.
Dix, M. R. & Hallpike, C. S. (1952) The pathology, symptomatology and diagnosis of certain common disorders of the vestibular system. *Proceedings of the Royal Society of Medicine,* **45,** 341-354.
Eviator, A. (1972) Interpretation of electronystagmographic results. *Laryngoscope,* **82,** 1059-1067.
Friedman, A. P., Brenner, C. & Denny-Brown, D. (1945) Post traumatic vertigo and dizziness. *Journal of Neurosurgery,* **2,** 36-41.
Fernandez, C. & Lindsay, J. R. (1960) Positional nystagmus in man and animals. *Journal of Nervous and Mental Disease,* **130,** 488-495.
Gayral, L. & Neuwirth, E. (1954) Oto-neuro-opthalmolgic manifestations of cervical origin. *New York State Medical Journal,* **54,** 1920-1926.
Glaser, M. (1937) The cause of dizziness in head injuries: vestibular test study in sixty-six patients. *Annals of Otology,* **46,** 387-392.
Gordon, N. (1954) Post traumatic vertigo. *Lancet,* **i,** 1216-1218.
Grove, W. E. (1928) Otologic observations in trauma of the head. *Archives of Otolaryngology,* **8,** 249-256.
Hall, J. (1679) *Select Observations on English Bodies* (Observation II; second century). London: J. Sherly.
Harrison, M. S. (1956) Notes on the clinical features and pathology of post traumatic vertigo with a special reference to positional nystagmus. *Brain,* **79,** 474-482.
Harrison, M. S. & Ozsahinoglu, C. (1972) Positional vertigo: aetiology and clinical significance. *Brain,* **95,** 369-372.

Hood, J. D. (1968) Electronystagmography. *Journal of Laryngology and Otology,* **82,** 67-183.

Hough, J. V. D. (1970) Fractures of the temporal bone and associated middle and inner ear trauma. *Proceedings of the Royal Society of Medicine,* **63,** 245-252.

Hough, J. V. D. & Stewart, W. D. (1968) Middle ear injuries in skull trauma. *Laryngoscope,* **78,** 899-937.

Jackson, R. (1966) *The Cervical Syndrome.* Springfield, Illinois: C. C. Thomas.

Jacobson, S. A. (1963) *The Post Traumatic Syndrome Following Head Injury.* Springfield, Illinois: C. C. Thomas.

Jongkees, L. B. W. (1969) Cervical vertigo. *Laryngoscope,* **79,** 1483-1484.

Jongkees, L. B. W. & Philipszoon, A. J. (1963) Electronystagmography. *Acta Oto-laryngologica.* Supplement 189.

Laszlo, I. (1973) Conventional radiography of the temporal bone *Otolaryngologic Clinics of North America,* **6,** 323-335.

Lieou, J. C. (1928) *Syndrome Sympathique Cervicale Posterieur et Arthrite Cervicale Chronique.* Strasbourg: These.

Linthicum, F. H. & Rand, C. W. (1931) Neuro-otologic observations in concussion of the brain. *Archives of Oto-laryngology,* **13,** 785-821.

Matthews, W. B. (1963) *Practical Neurology.* Oxford: Blackwell Scientific Publications.

Mathog, R. H. (1971) Temporal bone preparation by intra labyrinthine perfusion. *Archives of Oto-laryngology,* **93,** 610-614.

Ménière, P. (1861) Memoire sur des lésions de l'oreille intern donnant lieu à des symptomes de congestion cerebrale apoplectiforme. *Gazette Medicale de Paris,* **16,** 597-598.

Mygind, S. H. (1918) Traumatic vestibular diseases. *Acta Oto-laryngologica,* **1,** 515-531.

Nylen, C. O. (1950) Positional nystagmus; a review and future prospects. *Journal of Laryngology and Otology,* **64,** 205-218.

Osnato, M. & Gillibertini, V. (1927) Post concussion neurosis — traumatic encephalitis. A conception of post concussion phenomena. *Archives of Neurology and Psychiatry,* **18,** 181-211.

Passow, K. A. (1905) *Die Verletzungen des Gehorrobgames.* Munich: J. F. Bergmann.

Phillips, D. G. (1945) Investigation of vestibular function after head injury. *Journal of Neurology, Neurosurgery and Psychiatry,* **8,** 79-100.

Potter, G. D. (1972) Temporal bone fractures — problems in radiologic diagnosis. *Laryngoscope,* **82,** 408-413.

Preber, L. & Silfverskiöld, B. P. (1957) Paroxysmal positional vertigo following head injury. *Acta Oto-laryngologica,* **48,** 255-265.

Proctor, B., Gurdjian, E. S. & Webster, J. E. (1956) The ear in head trauma. *Laryngoscope,* **66,** 16-59.

Risk, E. J. E. (1890) A case of traumatic injury to the labyrinth of the right ear successfully treated with injections of Pilocarpine. *British Medical Journal,* **i,** 234-235.

Rowe, M. J. & Carlson, C. (1980) Brainstem auditory evoked potentials in post-concussion dizziness. *Archives of Neurology,* **37,** 679-683.

Rubin, W. (1969) Electronystagmography. *Archives of Oto-laryngology,* **89,** 45-47.

Russell, W. R. (1932) Cerebral involvement in head injury. A study based on the examination of 200 cases. *Brain,* **55,** 549-603.

Ryan, G. M. S. & Cope, S. (1955) Cervical vertigo. *Lancet,* **ii,** 1355-1357.

Schaller, W. F. (1939) After effects of head injury. *Journal of the American Medical Association,* **113,** 1779-1784.

Schuknecht, J. F. & Davison, R. C. (1956) Deafness and vertigo after head injury. *Archives of Oto-laryngology,* **63,** 513-528.

Schuknecht, J. F. (1969) The mechanism of inner ear injury from blows to the head. *Annals of Otology,* **78,** 253-262.

Schuster, F. B. (1927) Head injuries with ear symptoms. *South Western Medical Journal,* **11,** 116-122.

Silfverskiöld, B. P. (1969) The post concussional syndrome and its treatment. *The Late Effects of Head Injury* (Ed.) Walker, A. E., Caveness, W. F. & Critchley, M. Chapter 12. Springfield, Illinois: C. C. Thomas.

Steffen, T. N. (1965) Positional vertigo of traumatic origin relieved by section of the vestibular nerve. *Southern Medical Journal,* **58,** 587-592.

Strauss, S. F. & Savitsky, N. (1934) Head injuries: neurologic and psychiatric aspects. *Archives of Neurology and Psychiatry,* **31,** 893-955.

Symonds, C. P. (1942) Discussion on differential diagnosis and treatment of post concussional states. *Proceedings of the Royal Society of Medicine,* **35,** 25-38.

Taylor, A. R. (1967) Post concussional sequelae. *British Medical Journal,* **ii,** 67-70.

Taylor, A. R. & Bell, T. K. (1966) Slowing of cerebral circulation after concussional head injury. *British Medical Journal,* **ii,** 178-180.

Toglia, J. U. (1969) Dizziness after whiplash injury of the neck and closed head injury: electro-nystagmographic correlations. In *The Late Effects of Head Injury* (Ed.) Walker, A. E., Caveness, W. F. & Critchley, M. Chapter 6. Springfield, Illinois: C. C. Thomas.

Toglia, J. U. (1972) Vestibular and medico-legal aspects of closed craniocervical trauma. Electro-nystagmographic analysis of 568 patients. *Scandinavian Journal of Rehabilitation Medicine,* **4,** 126-132.

Toglia, J. U., Rosenberg, P. E. & Ronis, M. L. (1970) Post traumatic dizziness, vestibular, audiological and medicolegal aspects. *Archives of Oto-laryngology,* **92,** 845-892.

Tomlinson, B. E. (1970) Brain stem lesions after head injury. *Journal of Clinical Pathology,* **23,** (Supplement) *Royal College of Pathologists,* **4,** 154-165.

Windle, W. R., Groat, R. A. & Fox, C. A. (1944) Experimental structural alterations in the brain during and after concussion. *Surgery, Gynaecology and Obstetrics,* **79,** 561-584.

CHAPTER ELEVEN

The Postconcussional Syndrome

The discussion of post-traumatic headache and post-traumatic dizziness in the last two chapters inevitably leads to consideration of the so-called postconcussional syndrome. Without doubt a great many patients do complain of a variety of symptoms after head injury, often over prolonged periods of time. Headache and dizziness are the most common, but others such as impairment of memory, lack of concentration, irritability, fatigue, depression and alcohol intolerance also occur. Whilst it is convenient to gather these symptoms together when they coexist under the general heading of the post-concussional syndrome, the question as to whether they do in fact cluster with sufficient frequency and with sufficient constancy of pattern to justify such a label. Furthermore, does the concept of a specific syndrome help in the management of individual patients or in the understanding of the mechanisms underlying the development of these often disabling symptoms? One of our objectives in planning a longitudinal study of patients surviving head injury was to see if there were any factors: social, environmental, constitutional, or relating to the injury itself, which had special relevance to the development of the syndrome. Our hopes have not been completely fulfilled, but the experience of the study has led us to some tentative conclusions, which we offer for consideration.

Just how and when the term 'postconcussional syndrome' came into being is not certain, but it was probably first used by Strauss and Savitsky in 1934. Other names such as 'minor contusion syndrome' have been used, but they too have referred to this same group of symptoms that it has been found convenient to congregate under a somewhat vague umbrella term. There has been a good deal of uncertainty and often controversy about the nature of the syndrome — due in part at least to the variable basis on which studies of its nature and pathogenesis have been conducted. Head injury populations on which surveys have been based have tended to vary widely in their selection. The majority have been derived from hospital series, but in some instances the approach has been neurological and in others psychiatric and some studies have in fact emerged from medicolegal practice. There have also been wide differences in methods of follow-up and assessment, and discrepancies have arisen because of the varying intervals after injury at which surveys have been carried out.

PREVIOUS STUDIES

The Industrial Revolution brought in its wake a great increase in the number of accidental injuries, and the problem of persisting symptoms after injury soon came to light. Baron Dupuytren (1839) gave one of the earliest descriptions of the somatic and psychological consequences of head injury. Another early landmark was the publication by Erichsen in 1886 of a book entitled *On Concussion of the Spine, Nervous Shock and Other Obscure Injuries to the Nervous System*. He described 53 patients with severe injuries and concluded that the deficits he observed were due to 'molecular disarrangement'. In many ways his studies were inadequate; for instance he was unable to distinguish between disease of the spinal cord and disease of the brain. Nevertheless, Erichsen's studies are of historical importance in that they expressed a clear opinion in favour of an organic cause for the symptoms that follow central nervous system injury.

Even in those early days, opinion as to the nature of the common postconcussional symptoms became divided. Regler (1879) noted an increase in the amount of invalidism following railway accidents that seemed to coincide with the passage of the Compensation Law in 1871. He believed that the psychological impact of the accident itself and the shock and terror associated with it were important factors in influencing the long-term outcome. He thought that the protracted idleness that often followed injury and also the prospect of monetary gain played their part in perpetuating postinjury symptoms. Regler's views were largely supported by Strümpell (1888), who contrasted the sequelae of head injury with those following trauma to other parts of the body. He emphasized the tendency of patients following head injury to exaggerate their symptoms and, like Regler, attached considerable significance to the role of compensation in their perpetuation.

Oppenheim (1892) adopted a middle-of-the-road course in his description of the variety of clinical states that result from accidental injuries. He introduced the term 'traumatic neurosis' and included in this category all those neuropsychiatric sequelae of injury that could not be classified as hysteria or neurasthenia and that did not fall into any recognizable organic pattern. He suggested that it was the combination of organic and psychological factors that was responsible for traumatic neurosis, and it came to be regarded by many of his contemporaries as a new disease. Another early reference was that of Friedmann (1892). He emphasized the association of headache and dizziness with the other postconcussional symptoms already referred to and adopted the view that the whole constellation comprised a special syndrome which he called 'the vasomotor symptom complex' and which he believed to be due to 'disordered intracranial circulation'.

Despite advances in neurology and neurosurgery in the present century, including a greatly increased knowledge of the mechanisms and management of head injury, not much progress has been made in the understanding of the postconcussional syndrome. Controversies over its aetiology continue unabated. Every now and again they lead to interesting verbal confrontations and one such that involved the giants of the day is recorded in the Proceedings of the 46th Annual Meeting of the American Neurological Association in New York in 1920. Charles Dana (1920) of Cornell University Medical College presented an account of what he called 'traumatic conduct disorders'. He expressed profound scepticism as to their organic nature. The opposite view was vigorously upheld by Harvey Cushing who believed that, in spite of the absence of physical signs, generalized complaints following head injury were attributable to organic brain damage leading to permanent intellectual and occupational disablement. Francis Dercum, Bernard Sachs and Foster Kennedy disagreed with Cushing and generally supported Charles Dana. In retrospect it seems likely that Cushing's views were based on an experience of the more serious categories of head injury, but it is an interesting commentary on the continuing controversy that the same differences of opinion were being expressed fifty years later at a meeting of the Association of British Neurologists in Newcastle.

The increased number of head injuries occurring in war time and the special provision made for their management afforded opportunity for the study of the post-traumatic sequelae. Symonds (1942) made important observations on the variable patterns of the individual symptoms comprising the postconcussional syndrome. He recognized the different types of headache that patients complained of, and also noted that it was not uncommon for the onset of headache to be delayed. His view of the aetiology of postconcussional symptoms was that they were basically due to organic cerebral damage, but that the symptomatic expression of that damage was likely to be conditioned by psychological reaction. He wrote as follows: 'As to the distinction between the physiogenic and the psychogenic factors in a given case, they appear in most cases so closely intertwined that to separate them is unnatural. I am thinking, of course, of the case in which there is no doubt that organic cerebral damage has occurred. That a man with a hurt brain should have a disturbed mind is to be expected. It is equally to be expected that this disturbance will affect his capacity for adjustment as a whole. What then follows must depend upon the psychological situations to which adjustment is called for. The disorder of function is related not merely to any set task of the moment, but a continuous series of adjustments. This is why our formal psychiatric tests are of relatively little value in assessing disability. We need to get inside the man as far as possible, looking back into his past and forward into his future. Even so, it is often impossible to measure disability except by putting a man to his old occupation for a continuous period of some weeks and seeing what transpires.

'It will be understood from what I have said that I regard the practice of dividing the post-contusional cases into two groups, labelling the one organic and the other functional, or neurotic, as unprofitable and misleading.'

Denny-Brown (1943) held similar views to those of Symonds, although he believed that the postconcussional syndrome could occasionally occur as a pure psychoneurosis following a trivial head injury. He thought that true malingering was rare. A more recent study from New Zealand (Gronwall and Wrightson, 1974) has produced evidence that again would support the views expressed by Symonds. The authors believe that the syndrome begins on the basis of slightly impaired intellectual function resulting from organic brain damage. They argue that those in whom this minimal abnormality persists are prone to loss of confidence and to the development of psychoneurotic symptoms. The neurotic reaction may become fixed and may persist long after the cognitive defect is no longer demonstrable. The psychological studies of Dikmen and Reitan (1977) provide some support for this theory; they indicate that patients with initial and residual neuropsychological deficits show evidence of greater emotional distress than do patients without such deficits.

There is quite a lot of support for the theory that the postconcussional syndrome is purely psychogenic. Charcot repeatedly emphasized the latent interval that commonly occurs between injury and onset of symptoms and, believing strongly in the neurotic theory of causation, he termed this the 'period of meditation'. He was unequivocal in his view that the symptoms were due to hysteria and neurasthenia. Kay, Kerr and Lassman (1971) reached similar conclusions on the basis of their studies of 474 patients who had suffered head injuries. Those with postconcussional syndromes did not appear to have had more severe injuries than the others; they were distinguished from patients who did not have the syndrome principally on the basis of psychosocial factors. They tended to be in the middle age groups, to be married, to belong to social class 4, to have suffered an industrial accident, to be engaged in semiskilled occupations and to have had a previous psychiatric history.

There are also those who believe that the postconcussional syndrome not only lacks an organic basis but is due to frank malingering. Miller, in the Milroy Lectures which he gave to the Royal College of Physicians of London in 1961, advanced in forthright terms the view that patients with postconcussional syndromes were simulating or at least consciously exaggerating their symptoms. In his own case studies he established a relationship between the occurrence of the syndrome and the incidence of claims for compensation. Furthermore, he noted that the syndrome was more severe and more persistent in patients with minor head injuries, and he was struck by the absence of the syndrome as a sequel to sporting injuries. Cook (1969, 1972) has supported Miller's view and has demonstrated that patients with compensation claims tend to have a greater duration of symptoms and a longer absence from work than those without.

In summary, four main explanations for the postconcussional syndrome have been consistently advanced over the years. Each theory has been supported by carefully reasoned argument and also by detailed case study. The theories may be summarized as follows:

1. The organic theory — supported by those who believe that there is invariably some structural damage to brain substance.
2. Organic/psychological theory — assumes that there is always some organic damage; the manifestations in intellectual terms may be minimal, but are nevertheless of sufficient degree to lead to a psychoneurotic reaction when the individual is stressed.
3. Psychological/neurotic theory — visualizes a purely psychoneurotic basis without any organic substrate.
4. Theory of malingering — shares with (3) above the belief that there is no organic basis. But, in contrast to theory (3), it postulates a powerful element of conscious motivation which in many instances is related to prospects of monetary gain. To some extent the distinction between theories (3) and (4) reflects the differing views that exist on the psychodynamics of hysteria.

Against this background we analysed the data derived from our study, in the hope that its longitudinal structure might provide some additional evidence, but also in the belief that where four aetiological theories have survived for more than a century it is likely that each is applicable at least in a proportion of cases.

THE NEWCASTLE STUDY

It can be said at the outset that in the course of the study there were remarkably few occasions when 'the postconcussional syndrome' seemed an appropriate clinical diagnosis. The proformas on which all our data were recorded did not include reference to the syndrome as such, but routine hospital records were kept and letters were sent to family doctors and seldom if ever was the label of postconcussional syndrome attached. Indeed, it is not a term that the authors incline to use in their routine clinical practice.

Having declared our prejudice, let us look at the data objectively to see if they tell

Table 11.1. Patients' symptoms on discharge and at follow-up (Newcastle series).

	Discharge	6 months	1 year	2 years
Total number of patients	372	338	323	300
Headache	135	91	58	72
Dizziness	72	74	45	54
Depression	31	60	58	56
Anxiety	30	40	45	48
Impairment of concentration	14	21	32	33
Impairment of memory	7	20	28	31
Irritability	3	31	23	17
Fatigue	12	14	18	17
Decreased alcohol tolerance	0	7	6	5
Blackouts	3	5	6	4
Loss of drive	1	4	4	3
Hypersensitivity to noise	0	4	3	3
Light sensitivity	2	3	2	2
Incompetence	1	2	1	2
Loss of libido	0	2	1	1
Absence of emotion	0	2	1	1
Increased alcohol tolerance	0	1	1	0
Impotence	0	1	1	0

us anything about the concept of the syndrome. Table 11.1 lists all the symptoms which might be included among its constituent elements. It is based mainly on the psychiatric symptom check list that was used, but there were also inputs from other parts of the data bank. The table shows the numbers of patients in whom each symptom was noted to be present at the time of discharge and at each of the follow-up visits. The numbers recorded include all patients who mentioned each particular symptom whether spontaneously or in response to general or direct questioning. It will be seen that headache leads the field by a substantial margin. Dizziness comes second, with a figure about 20 per cent lower, except at the time of discharge when the incidence of dizziness is just over half that of headache. In both instances there is a decline in incidence over successive follow-up periods, except for an interesting upturn at two years. After headache and dizziness come depression and anxiety, each with a high incidence, the former being slightly more common than the latter except at the time of discharge, when numbers are about equal. In contrast to headache and dizziness, there is a higher incidence of depression and anxiety at follow-up than at the time of discharge and there there is little fluctuation in the figures throughout the follow-up period.

The next group of symptoms with roughly comparable levels of incidence includes impairment of concentration, impairment of memory, irritability and fatigue. The first two show a gradual increase in frequency at successive follow-up intervals, in contrast to headache and dizziness which, as noted previously, had the opposite trend except at two years. Irritability has a temporal pattern very like that of depression, whilst fatigue, which was complained of rather less frequently than might have been expected, remains at a fairly constant level throughout. Next in rank order, but at a much lower incidence level, come alcohol intolerance and blackouts, nearly all of which were post-traumatic seizures. Finally, at the bottom of the league there are a variety of symptoms which occur with negligible frequency and could scarcely qualify for inclusion in the syndrome.

The figures in Table 11.1 pick out clearly those particular symptoms which so commonly persist after head injury and confirm what has been said many times before. The incidence figures are high, but this reflects to some extent our method of scoring. It will be remembered that patients whose complaints were elicited only on direct questioning were included along with those who volunteered them spontaneously. Table 11.2 also lists the main symptoms, but the figures relate only to patients who offered them of their own accord without prompting. This method of scoring reduces the figures and brings them more in line with those reported recently by Rutherford, Merrett and McDonald (1978). It evens out some of the serial changes noted in Table 11.1 and it brackets depression along with headache and dizziness as a leading postconcussional symptom.

Table 11.2. Patients with spontaneous symptoms on discharge and at follow-up (Newcastle series).

	Discharge	6 months	1 year	2 years
Total number of patients	372	338	323	300
Headache	79	30	15	6
Dizziness	34	26	6	6
Depression	7	11	12	11
Anxiety	6	7	6	6
Impairment of concentration	8	3	3	4
Impairment of memory	4	4	1	2
Irritability	0	5	7	3
Fatigue	1	3	4	3
Decreased alcohol tolerance	0	0	0	0
Blackouts	0	1	1	1

Taken at their face value, the data in these tables would seem to imply that a considerable number of patients after head injury do complain of a group of symptoms, headache and dizziness being chief amongst them, that can appropriately be subsumed under the traditional heading of the postconcussional syndrome. The syndrome concept, implying a 'going together' of a number of symptoms, would seem to be justified. But on returning to some of the tables in the chapter on headache (Tables 9.8, 9.17—19), in which headache is related to other major postconcussional symptoms at discharge and at each of the follow-up periods, we find that those symptoms, whilst occurring more frequently in patients with headache, nevertheless are well represented in the group without headache. So too if we look at other individual symptoms and relate them to the major post-concussional items, we find that clustering is less consistent than might have been expected and that, furthermore, the numerical relationship between the major symptoms varies at the different stages of follow-up.

To pursue this line of enquiry further, let us look at headache itself in greater detail. It will be remembered that the longitudinal nature of the study revealed that, in the follow-up period, patients with headache fell into two categories: those whose headache originated at the time of the injury and persisted during the follow-up period (persisting headache), and those who developed headache in the course of follow-up (late-acquired headache). In Table 11.3, the numbers of patients in the two categories of headache and of those without any headache are related to the frequency of dizziness, depression and anxiety at the various follow-up periods. Whilst at six months dizziness is equally common in the two headache categories, at one and two years it is distinctly more common in patients with the early-onset, persisting type of headache. This is not so in the case of depression and anxiety, which at all follow-up periods are less common in those with early-onset headache than in those with late-acquired headache. Indeed those two symptoms are not much more frequent in the group with early-onset headache than in patients with no headache at all.

Table 11.3. Headache in relation to other postconcussional symptoms (Newcastle series).

		Dizziness		Depression		Anxiety		Total patients
		No.	(%)	No.	(%)	No.	(%)	
6 months	Headache:							
	Early onset	24	48	6	12	6	12	50
	Late onset	20	49	18	44	12	29	41
	None	30	12	36	15	22	9	247
1 year	Headache:							
	Early onset	12	41	6	21	5	17	29
	Late onset	4	14	9	31	10	34	29
	None	29	11	43	16	30	11	265
2 years	Headache:							
	Early onset	17	46	8	22	5	14	37
	Late onset	10	29	12	34	11	31	35
	None	27	12	36	16	32	14	228

When dizziness is broken down into early-onset and late-onset categories (Table 11.4), we find an almost identical incidence of headache in both categories, and this applies at all follow-up periods. As was the case with headache, the late-onset variety of dizziness was associated with higher rates of depression and anxiety than was the early-onset variety. Also, as was discussed in Chapter 10, patients in the latter category proved less likely to process claims for compensation.

The relationship between headache and dizziness may be pursued further by comparing the incidence figures in the different breakdown categories (Table 11.5). This shows the figures at the six-month follow-up and illustrates that patients with early-onset dizziness, which is so often associated with positional nystagmus, are highly likely to suffer from headache; this in the majority of cases will be of the late acquired variety. Indeed, of the 33 patients with early onset of dizziness only 13 had no complaint of headache at six months, and exactly the same number were complaining of late acquired headache. Looking at the patients with persisting headache, we find that half of them were complaining of dizziness at six months, but in the majority of cases this was of the late acquired variety; it was unlikely therefore to be accompanied by positional nystagmus as proof of an organic cause.

Table 11.4. Dizziness in relation to other postconcussional symptoms (Newcastle series).

		Headache		Depression		Anxiety		Total patients
		No.	(%)	No.	(%)	No.	(%)	
6 months	Dizziness:							
	Early onset	20	60	4	12	2	6	33
	Late onset	24	59	16	39	10	24	41
	None	47	18	40	15	28	11	264
1 year	Dizziness:							
	Early onset	9	36	4	16	1	4	25
	Late onset	7	35	7	35	4	20	20
	None	42	15	47	17	40	14	278
2 years	Dizziness:							
	Early onset	11	50	5	23	4	18	22
	Late onset	16	50	14	44	4	13	32
	None	45	18	37	15	40	16	246

Table 11.5 Headache and dizziness at six months (Newcastle series).

	Headache			
	Early onset	Late onset	None	*Total*
Dizziness:				
Early onset	7	13	13	*33*
Late onset	17	7	17	*41*
None	26	21	217	*264*
Total	*50*	*41*	*247*	*338*

Cross-comparisons between the various symptoms we have studied can obviously be pursued at great length and what invariably emerges is that there is variability and inconstancy in numerical relationships that are concealed by straightforward summations. The point is brought out most clearly by examining separately the correlations of early-onset and late-onset symptoms. On the basis of headache and dizziness figures along we can recognize three quite distinct groups of patients: those with an early onset of one symptom who go on during the follow-up period to develop the other; those who at discharge have neither headache nor dizziness and subsequently acquire both; and those who have both headache and dizziness at discharge and in whom both symptoms persist into the follow-up period. The more symptoms we incorporate in the concatenation the more apparent does the heterogeneity of the postconcussional syndrome become.

CONCLUSIONS

A number of points arise from this study which make us question the validity of the concept of a postconcussional syndrome. The recognition that one of the principal constituents, namely dizziness, is in some cases clearly organic and in others almost certainly not, underlines the widely differing disorders that may exist in patients to whom the same diagnostic label is attached. We have already emphasized the fact that a patient with headache may be in the process of recovering from something that has affected him since the time of his head injury or, on the other hand, he may equally well be in the early stages of development of a late acquired headache, and that the implications will be strikingly different with regard to probable associations with other symptoms. The figures derived from the study bear out our clinical impression that depression is a factor of major importance in a great many patients with symptoms after head injury. This is scarcely to be wondered at when one thinks of the psychological impact of accidents, which are so often frightening and demoralizing and almost invariably associated with worry or unhappiness of one sort or another. To be knocked down by a motor car can be as shocking as a bereavement for an elderly person. It is our belief that in a great many patients the symptoms ascribed to the so-called postconcussional syndrome are in fact the physical manifestations of a true reactive depression.

We have already discussed the way in which correlations between the symptoms vary at the different follow-up intervals and we believe that this in some cases reflects a causal relationship. We would contend that in most instances where the term syndrome aids us in our appreciation of a disease process, the several components are juxtaposed in a relatively consistent manner, but that this condition certainly does not apply in the case of the postconcussional syndrome.

It is therefore suggested that there is so much variation in the nature of the constituents of the postconcussional syndrome and so much inconstancy in their inter-relationships that the term distracts us from a proper analysis of the true nature of the patient's complaints and invites us to lump together a great many differing disorders under a single diagnostic umbrella. This carries the added risk that a single aetiological mechanism may be assumed; perhaps this is why there has been so much controversy over the nature of the syndrome.

Earlier in the chapter we summarized the four main theories of causation of the postconcussional syndrome and we referred to the proponents of each. We would contend that the syndrome itself was misconceived and that the search for a unitary hypothesis was therefore ill-fated. Indeed we believe that all four of the suggested mechanisms operate in the production of postconcussional symptoms. None would doubt the organic nature of the complaints in some patients and the demonstration of positional nystagmus argues most strongly for the existence of structural damage in some with dizziness. We would also accept without reservation the notion that, in many patients, the postconcussional symptoms have both organic and psychological causes. We believe, for instance, that the frequent development of late acquired headache in patients with early-onset dizziness strongly supports this theory. Nor would we doubt that in a number of patients, particularly those who have suffered minor head injuries, the subsequent symptoms may be entirely psychological in origin, with no suggestion at all of structural damage to skull or brain. Perhaps the most common group in this category are those patients who develop a depression as a result of their accident.

Finally, what of malingering? In our experience, true conscious malingering for financial or other personal gain is a rare phenomenon. However, it clearly does occur, and Miller (1961) has provided indisputable examples. But neurologists vary widely in their interpretation of physical signs which cannot be attributed to structural disease. Every experienced neurologist is familiar with the leg that has satisfactorily hoisted its owner on to the examination couch yet has failed to rise three inches from the couch in formal tests of hip flexion; or the brawny forearm whose flexor and extensor muscles are in such conflict that the grip is reduced to quivering incompetence. In the context of medicolegal examination these performances are apt to be attributed to attempted deception for the basest of motives, yet how often are they encountered in everyday practice, where 'functional overlay' is readily accepted on the basis of anxiety or diminished expectation of performance in a genuinely impaired member.

We would therefore like to see an acceptance of the fact that postconcussional symptoms are varied in their nature, their causation and their interdependence. We would urge that each one should be analysed in detail and assessed on its merits, bearing particularly in mind its time of onset in relation to the injury if this can be established. We believe that, in the interests both of patients who have suffered head injuries and of our understanding of the nature of their symptoms, we should abandon the concept of the postconcussional syndrome and the controversies that surround it.

REFERENCES

Cook, J. B. (1969) The effects of minor head injuries sustained in sport and the post concussional syndrome. In *The Late Effects of Head Injury*. (Ed.) Walker, A. E., Caveness, W. F. & Critchley, M. pp. 408-413. Springfield, Illinois: C. C. Thomas.

Cook, J. B. (1972) The post concussional syndrome and factors influencing recovery after minor head injury admitted to hospital. *Scandinavian Journal of Rehabilitation Medicine,* **4,** 27-30.

Dana, C. L. (1920) Wounds of the head and compensation laws. *Archives of Neurology and Psychiatry,* **4,** 479-483.

Denny-Brown, D. (1943) Post-concussion syndrome — a critique. *Annals of Internal Medicine,* **19,** 427-432.

Dikmen, S. & Reitan, R. M. (1977) Emotional sequelae of head injury. *Annals of Neurology,* **2,** 492-494.

Dupuytren, G. (1839) *Lecons Orales de Clinique Chirurgicale Faites a L'Hotel — Dieu de Paris.* Edition 2 Volume 5. Paris: Germer-bailliere.

Erichsen, J. D. (1886) *On Concussion of the Spine, Nervous shock and other Obscure Injuries to the Nervous System.* New Edition. Baltimore: William Wood.

Friedmann, M. (1892) Uber eine besondere schwere Form von Folgezustandes nach Gehirnerschutterung und uber den vasomotorischen Symptomen Complex bei derselben im Allgemeinen. *Archiv Für Psychiatrie,* **23,** 230-238.

Gronwall, D. & Wrightson, P. (1974) Delayed recovery of intellectual function after minor head injury. *Lancet,* **ii,** 605-609.

Kay, D. W. K., Kerr, T. A. & Lassman, L. P. (1971) Brain trauma and the post concussional syndrome. *Lancet,* **ii,** 1052-1055.

Miller, H. (1961) Accident neurosis. *British Medical Journal,* **i,** 919-925, 992-998.

Oppenheim, H. (1892) Die traumatischen Neurosen nach den Verletzung. In *Der Nervenklinik Der Charite In Den 8 Jarhren* (1883-1891) Edited 1. Berlin: A. Hirschwald.

Regler, J. (1879) *Uber die Folgen der Verletzung auf Eisenbahnen insbesonder der Verletzungen des Ruchenmarks.* Berlin: G. Reimer.

Rutherford, W. H., Merrett, J. D. & McDonald, J. R. (1978) Symptoms at one year following concussion from minor head injuries. *Injury,* **10,** 225-230.

Strumpell, A. (1888) *Uber die Traumatischen Neurosen.* Berlin: Gustav Fischer.

Strauss, I. & Savitsky, N. (1934) Head injury: Neurologic and psychiatric aspects. *Archives of Neurology and Psychiatry,* **31,** 893-954.

Symonds, C. P. (1942) Discussion on differential diagnosis and treatment of post-contusional states. *Proceedings of the Royal Society of Medicine,* **35,** 601-607.

CHAPTER TWELVE

The Medical Sequelae of Head Injury

The purpose of this chapter is to review some of the disturbances following head injury that may affect systems other than the nervous system. It is common practice for patients with head injury to be cared for in specialized neurosurgical units and it is important for those people who are normally preoccupied with disorders of the nervous system to be alert to the signs of disorder in other systems. In the next chapter we shall emphasize the need to recognize injuries in sites such as the thorax or abdomen as being potential causes of cerebral dysfunction. Here the opposite problem is being considered; that is, where damage to the brain can cause disorders, often subtle ones, in distant regions or systems. All the conditions to be considered are uncommon and few are represented in the Newcastle study.

THE METABOLIC EFFECTS OF HEAD INJURY

There is an extensive literature on the subject of metabolic response to injury. Most studies have been concerned with the effects of whole body injury rather than of injury to the head alone. Such studies of the latter as have been undertaken have failed to identify any metabolic response that is specific to head injury. One of the difficulties in this field is, of course, to dissect out the effects of head injury from those due to blood loss, starvation, emotion, pain, shock, or drugs and anaesthetic agents. The changes in electrolytes, proteins and glucose homeostasis that occur after trauma generally (Wright, 1979) undoubtedly occur in patients who have suffered severe head injuries (Higgins et al, 1954). For a detailed account of the general metabolic effects of injury, the reader is referred to the excellent review by McLaurin and King (1975).

One aspect of metabolism which clearly can be disturbed selectively as a result of head injury is that associated with neuroendocrine function.

NEUROENDOCRINE DISORDERS AFTER HEAD INJURY

Pathology

Postmortem studies of patients dying as a result of head injury have shown that lesions of the pituitary and hypothalamus are much more common than might be supposed. Daniel, Pritchard and Treip (1959) first described acute infarction of the anterior lobe of the pituitary resulting from injury. In a later publication, Daniel and Treip (1961) described their finding of haemorrhage in the posterior lobe of the pituitary in just under 50 per cent of 152 consecutive fatal head injuries. In this series, small anterior lobe infarcts were also found in a few cases, and in eight patients there had been acute massive infarction of the anterior lobe. The authors suggested that infarction of the anterior lobe was due either to rupture of the pituitary stalk or to interruption of the hypophyseal portal vessels. Kornblum and Fisher (1969) studied 100 pituitary glands of patients who had died from craniocerebral injury, and they found lesions in 62. These included capsular haemorrhage, hypophyseal stalk haemorrhage, stalk laceration, posterior lobe infarction and ischaemic necrosis of the anterior lobe, which occurred in 22 of the cases. The most common lesion was haemorrhage into the capsule; this was noted in 56 of the glands studied.

Treip (1970) described changes in the hypothalamus as well as in the pituitary itself in patients dying as a result of head injury. Crompton (1971 and 1975) confirmed that hypothalamic lesions occur not uncommonly in fatal head injuries.

Clinical Manifestations of Hypothalmic and Pituitary Dysfunction

Despite the frequency of pathological changes in the hypothalamus and pituitary following head injury, clinical evidence of hypopituitarism is rare (Witter and Tascher, 1957). The most common endocrine disorder after head injury is undoubtedly diabetes insipidus (Porter and Miller, 1948). Its true incidence is difficult to estimate, but Porter and Miller (1948) reported 30 cases amongst approximately 5000 patients admitted to the Military Hospital for Head Injuries in Oxford. More recently Lewin, Marshall and Roberts (1979) have recorded eight cases in a consecutive series of 7000 patients admitted with head injury to the Regional Accident Service in Oxford. Diabetes insipidus is most likely to result from a severe head injury in which there is also damage to the olfactory nerves and the optic chiasma. It tends to recover spontaneously within a year of the injury.

Apart from classical diabetes insipidus, other disorders of salt and water metabolism may occur as a result of head injury. Golonka and Richardson (1970) described a patient who developed chronic serum hyperosmolality which was attributed to a loss of thirst perception after head injury. They suggested that there had been a change in the 'setting' of the osmoreceptors as a result of damage to the hypothalamus. Inappropriate antidiuretic hormone secretion, comparable to that seen with bronchial carcinoma, is another clinical syndrome that has been attributed to head injury. Two cases of this syndrome have been described in patients with subdural haematoma (Maroon and Campbell, 1970). The concept of primary cerebral hyponatraemia, at one time accepted as a possible consequence of head injury and of other cerebral disorders, was criticized by Ross and Christie (1969). They found it hard to accept and, amongst other things, argued that the osmoreceptors of an unconscious patient reside in the head of the attendant physician, who alone can ensure that water intake is adequate.

In the literature, there are surprisingly few reports of hypopituitarism resulting from head injury. When it does occur, it generally follows severe injury; the patients reported by Paxson and Brown (1976) and Winternitz (1976) had periods of post-traumatic amnesia in excess of 12 hours. By contrast, a single patient was reported (Altman and Pruzanski, 1961) in whom the head injury was said not even to have caused unconsiousness.

In addition to these cases of true hypopituitarism there are reports of a variety of hypothalamic disorders attributed to head injury. Byrne (1951) described a child aged four-and-a-half years who, following a relatively minor head injury, developed hyperphagia, excessive facial sweating, disordered temperature regulation and intermittent restlessness. Payne and De Wardener (1958) reported a 40-year-old male patient who had suffered a severe head injury with a post-traumatic amnesia of seven days, and who subsequently showed progressive weight gain. Ten years after the injury he showed a reversal of the normal diurnal urinary rhythm, with an output which was greater during the night than the day.

Binder and Gerstenbrand (1976) have reviewed various hypothalamic syndromes, some of them slightly controversial, which have been attributed to head injury. They refer to disturbances of thermoregulation and sweating, and emphasize their occurrence particularly in the acute stages after head injury. They describe also the disturbances of sleep rhythm and appetite that may follow severe head injury, and mention the occurrence of narcolepsy and of a condition akin to the Kleine—Levin syndrome. Lewin, Marshall and Roberts (1979), in their Oxford series, referred to 16 cases of hyperphagia amongst their total of 7000 patients with head injury.

Pituitary Function Studies in the Acute Stages after Head Injury

McLaurin and King (1975) reviewed the literature on pituitary function studies in relation to acute head injury. The last few years have seen a great many developments in endocrine biochemistry with the emergence of increasing numbers of highly sophisticated tests and, in retrospect, many of the studies referred to be McLaurin and King seem inadequate by present-day standards. Some depended on no more than serial estimations of circulating hormones. Thus King et al (1970) recorded only serial plasma cortisol levels. McCarthy et al (1964) employed the methopyrapone test in patients with acute head injury, but this particular test has largely been superseded. One reported study (Rudman et al, 1977) was based on a wide range of hormone estimations, including plasma levels of TSH, thyroxine, LH, FSH and testosterone. The evidence suggested that suprahypophyseal hypothyroidism and hypogonadism were common in patients who had suffered severe head injury with coma lasting for two or more weeks. It is to be hoped that more studies of this kind using up-to-date biochemical methods will be conducted.

The Newcastle Series

Some of the observations referred to in the foregoing sections were confirmed by the patients in the Newcastle study, even though detailed neuroendocrine tests were not performed routinely on all of them.

Case 71. This patient was thought probably to have features of a hypothalamic syndrome. She was a girl of 19 who was knocked down by a car. She was admitted initially to a local hospital in a semiconscious state but, as her condition deteriorated, she was transferred to the Newcastle General Hospital. At this time she was deeply unconscious, with fixed, dilated pupils, no spontaneous eye movements, absent oculocephalic reflexes and bilateral extensor motor responses, and decerebrate posturing. A left-sided extradural haematoma was removed. Recovery was slow; on discharge from hospital six weeks after the injury there was still evidence of a moderate dysphasia, profound intellectual impairment and bilateral pyramidal signs with only slight weakness but a marked increase in tone and reflexes. She did not menstruate for five months following the accident and, when seen at her six months' review, she was reported by her mother to have gained two stones in weight and to have a voracious appetite. By the end of two years her weight had returned to its preaccident level and her periods were regular. There was then no evidence of pituitary dysfunction, but she had a persisting personality change.

Two patients in the study developed diabetes insipidus. They were among the seven who had c.s.f. rhinorrhoea, and both had presumptive evidence of hypothalamic dysfunction.

Case 407. This patient was a 17-year-old boy who had a head injury as a result of a motorcycle accident. On admission to hospital he was unconscious and did not respond to spoken commands. He had a right frontal fracture which extended into the frontal sinus and within 24 hours he was noted to have CSF trickling from the right nostril. By this stage it was possible to make a rough assessment of his vision; it was obvious that it was grossly impaired. He had polyuria, with an output of up to six litres per day. His diabetes insipidus was controlled by injection of pitressin tannate in oil, but he underwent craniotomy 12 days after the accident because of persisting c.s.f. rhinorrhoea. Though this was successfully stopped he was left with bilateral anosmia, a bitemporal hemianopia, and vision in the left eye reduced to the appreciation of hand movements. Prolonged treatment of the diabetes insipidus was required, but the condition had resolved by the end of a year. However, during that period he had put on three stones in weight. He underwent extensive endocrine investigation but no abnormalities were demonstrated and, with dieting, he eventually returned to within a stone of his preaccident weight. His initial injury had been severe with post-traumatic amnesia in excess of two weeks.

Case 329. This patient was injured in a car accident and also had diabetes insipidus. He suffered a penetrating injury in the left frontal region and on admission he had a blood-stained watery nasal discharge. He was immediately taken to theatre because of the presence of a compound depressed fracture and he was found to have a frontal cerebral laceration and a dural tear, which was repaired. He was blind in his left eye and had diabetes insipidus with a urine output in excess of five litres. This was controlled adequately by lysine vasopressin nasal spray, which was required for only six days, following which there was spontaneous improvement. At the six-month follow-up his main complaint was of sleepiness which had not been present prior to the accident and for which he had been referred by his family doctor to a psychiatrist. The latter elicited a history of hypnagogic hallucinations as well as of sleepiness, but there was no history of cataplexy. However, the sleepiness was thought to be severe enough to justify a diagnosis of post-traumatic narcolepsy and the patient was treated with amphetamine. This was continued for four years but was then withdrawn. There were no late relapses of the sleepiness, but he was left with blindness in the left eye.

It has to be admitted that the evidence for hypothalamic—pituitary dysfunction in the above cases is somewhat tenuous and that the diagnoses are purely presumptive. However, since the study was completed, we have seen a patient with definite post-traumatic hypopituitarism.

This patient was a girl who fell from her bicycle and suffered a basal skull fracture with bleeding from the right ear. She appeared to make a good recovery, and the duration of post-traumatic amnesia was estimated at 48 hours. Prior to her accident she had menstruated regularly, but after it she developed oligomenorrhoea. Six months after the accident she was admitted to hospital in a confused state and was found to have a low serum sodium of 127 mmol/l and a plasma osmolality of 263 mosmol/kg. Over the space of two or three days her electrolytes returned to normal, her confusion resolved and she was discharged home. She was first seen in our department when she had a major convulsion some nine months after the original accident. There were no abnormalities on neurological examination, but the serum electrolytes were persistently abnormal, with low sodium and low plasma osmolality. Endocrine investigation showed normal levels of serum FSH and LH, low thyroxine at 50 nmol/l and a low TSH level at less than one mU/l. Her cortisol response to insulin-induced hypoglycaemia was poor. A six-and-a-half-hour water deprivation test (Dashe et al, 1963) for diabetes insipidus was normal. On the basis of these tests it was concluded that the head injury had resulted in partial pituitary failure with ACTH and TSH deficiency, as well as gonadotrophin deficiency as manifest by her oligomenorrhoea. She was given replacement therapy with hydrocortisone and thyroxine and at follow-up a year later she was well, with a normal menstrual pattern. Her endocrine tests were repeated and the findings were the same. It was concluded that she had persistent ACTH and TSH deficiency, but that gonadotrophin function had recovered. After a further two years she remains well, with normal menstruation and no further seizures.

Our limited experience in Newcastle of post-traumatic hypothalamic—pituitary dysfunction seems to conform to the generally accepted pattern. The most common disturbance is diabetes insipidus; this usually results from severe frontal injuries and frequently recovers spontaneously. Other hypothalamic disturbances resulting in altered sleep pattern or change in appetite may sometimes be encountered, but usually following only severe injuries. Detailed studies of pituitary function using the most up-to-date techniques have not been widely performed in patients who have had severe head injuries and it seems likely that they would reveal abnormalities that we are not at present detecting. This would certainly be our prediction, bearing in mind the high incidence of pathological change in the pituitary and hypothalamus of patients dying as the result of head injury.

CARDIOVASCULAR DISTURBANCES AFTER HEAD INJURY

The best-known vasomotor phenomenon that may be associated with acute head injury is the so-called 'Cushing response', in which a rising intracranial pressure is associated with a rising systemic blood pressure and a progressively slowing pulse rate. Other changes have been observed and many have been recorded in the German literature. The subject is well reviewed by Binder and Gerstenbrand (1976). Particular mention may be made of the report of Braun and Shoemaker (1973) who described a reduction in stroke volume and cardiac output combined with a marked tachycardia in patients with severe brain damage, and they noted a return to normal during the phase of recovery. They attributed these haemodynamic changes to disturbances of central regulatory mechanisms. It is common clinical experience that pulse and blood pressure show wide fluctuations in association with the decerebrate spasms of acute brain-stem injury. The changes may in fact be due to damage to the hypothalamus and they may be accompanied by other phenomena of similar origin, such as excessive sweating or temperature fluctuation (Woodhall, 1936).

Electrocardiographic abnormalities are well recognized in association with subarachnoid haemorrhage (de Swiet, 1969) and other types of intracranial haemorrhage (Weidler, 1974). They also occur after head injury. The most common changes are prolongation of the QT interval and increased voltage of the P wave. Other less frequent changes are increase in the QRS voltage and inversion of the T wave in the precordial leads (Hersch, 1961). The frequency with which electro-cardiographic changes occur in acutely brain-damaged patients is uncertain, but Julkunen et al (1972) have reported abnormalities in five out of a total of 165 injured patients treated in an intensive care unit. Little attempt seems to have been made so far to correlate electrocardiographic abnormalities with characteristics of the head injury, such as site and severity, and the prognostic significance of such changes is uncertain. A limited amount of experimental work on electrocardiographic changes following head injury in monkeys has been reported (Fernando et al, 1969).

The mechanisms whereby intracranial lesions produce electrocardiographic disturbances have always been a matter of speculation. Connor (1968) described a series of 231 autopsies on patients dying as a result of brain lesions. Twenty per cent of them had had head injuries. In 18 instances he was able to show definite histological abnormality in the myocardium, with foci of myocytolysis, usually in the left ventricle. The precise cause of such changes is unknown, but it has been suggested in the case of subarachnoid haemorrhage that changes in the hypothalamus result in high circulating catecholamine levels, which produce the cardiac lesions and the electrocardiographic abnormalities (Doshi and Neil-Dwyer, 1977). Presumably, similar mechanisms could operate in the case of head injury.

Newcastle Series

Included in the study were a number of patients who showed quite striking changes in blood pressure and pulse rate soon after their injuries, but they could generally be accounted for on the basis of injuries to other parts of the body.

One patient, a man aged 42 years, who was not eligible for inclusion in the study because he died 15 hours after his head injury, was thought to have neurogenic hypotension. On admission to hospital he was totally flaccid and had no eye-opening, vocal or motor response to pain. Corneal, pupillary, oculocephalic and oculovestibular reflexes were all absent and he had very irregular respiration, as a result of which he was put on a ventilator. From the time of admission his blood pressure remained exceedingly low, with a systolic reading of 60 mm Hg (7.9 kPa) and an unrecordable diastolic reading. He was anuric and, despite transfusions and the use of vasopressor agents, his blood pressure could not be restored. At autopsy there was no evidence of injury other than to the brain, which showed diffuse swelling and extensive frontal laceration. There was haemorrhage in the region of the pituitary but the stalk was intact. The heart was normal and no significant electrocardiographic abnormalities had been demonstrated prior to death.

GASTROINTESTINAL SEQUELAE OF HEAD INJURY

In 1772 John Hunter reported on the occurrence of gastric ulceration in two patients who had died as a result of head injury. Cushing (1932) gave a lucid description of ulcers in patients with brain injury and suggested a diencephalic cause for the hyperacidity to which he ascribed the ulcers. It is now recognized that all critically ill patients are susceptible to stress ulceration (Croker, 1979), and it is now widely accepted that H2 receptor antagonists should be employed in seriously ill patients thought to be at risk of gastrointestinal haemorrhage.

There is ample documentation of the increased gastric acid secretion thought to be responsible for stress ulcers. Watts and Clark (1969) showed that the highest levels of acid secretion were to be found in comatose patients with decerebrate rigidity. Idjadi et al (1971) not only showed high levels of gastric acid in patients with gastrointestinal bleeding following head injury but they also demonstrated increased pepsin secretion. They suggested too that a defect in the production of gastric mucus might be an additional factor in the causation of ulcers. Figures reflecting the frequency of stress ulceration in patients with head injury have varied; Watts and Clark (1970) thought that the incidence was as high as 60 per cent, whereas Norton, Greer and Eiseman (1970) reported a lower figure of 16 per cent.

On the evidence available it seems clear that in the acute stages after head injury unconscious patients, particularly those with decerebrate rigidity, have a significant risk of gastrointestinal haemorrhage. Although the results of controlled studies have not yet been published, it would seem reasonable to give prophylactic treatment with H2 receptor antagonists to these patients.

In the Newcastle series there were no cases of acute upper gastrointestinal haemorrhage, and no gastric ulcers or erosions were seen at autopsy in those patients who had died.

RESPIRATORY ABNORMALITIES AFTER HEAD INJURY

The act of breathing is achieved by the integration of neural influences originating at a variety of levels in the brain. It is not surprising that respiratory abnormalities occur commonly following head injury. Some of them were referred to in Chapter Six. A particularly useful contribution to our understanding of the neuropathological correlates of respiratory abnormalities was made by Plum and Posner (1972).

One of our patients, whose early death precluded admission to the Newcastle series, provided an example of a respiratory disorder that is commonly seen in patients with severe head injuries.

The patient was a man aged 37 who had had a fall at work. On admission to hospital he was deeply unconscious and was showing spontaneous decerebrate spasms. These continued for the next 12 hours. With each spasm there was a striking increase in the depth of his respiration, which would also become more rapid. As the spasm passed off, both the rate and depth of respiration would decrease. His condition deteriorated rapidly and, despite the removal of bilateral subdural haematomas, he died within 18 hours of admission. Autopsy showed severe and extensive brain damage.

We have emphasized already the importance of recognizing that respiratory disturbances in unconscious head-injury patients may simply be an expression of mechanical obstruction of the respiratory passages. Mendelson (1946) has drawn attention to the effects on the respiratory tract of aspiration of gastric acid. We have also mentioned the possibility that direct lung contusion and rib fractures may cause respiratory abnormalities; such injuries are easily overlooked in the setting of a head injury.

A respiratory abnormality about which there is considerable controversy is the so-called 'neurogenic pulmonary oedema', which is said to occur in a number of cases of acute head injury. The validity of the concept gains some support from experimental work in animals. Beckman and Bean (1969) were able to show that pulmonary oedema developed in 92 per cent of rats subjected to head injury so severe as to be almost instantaneously fatal. They subsequently showed that monkeys subjected to head injury developed reduced pulmonary compliance which could be prevented by pretreatment with Dibenzyline, suggesting that the sympathetic nervous system played a part in the production of the pulmonary abnormality (Beckman, Bean and Baslock, 1971). There is also clinical evidence in support of the view that neurogenic pulmonary oedema occurs in man. Ducker (1968) suggested that it developed only in those with increased intracranial pressure. On the basis of experience with Vietnam combat casualties, Simmons et al (1969) reported that autopsies carried out on soldiers dying from head injuries showed that the majority had pulmonary oedema. The phenomenon was noted even in casualties dying within minutes of the injury.

Theories of the pathogenesis of neurogenic pulmonary oedema have been reviewed by Theodore and Robin (1975). The difficulty, of course, is to exclude the possibility that the pulmonary oedema is the result of aspiration of foreign material into the lungs. In the Newcastle series, a number of patients dying from their head injuries were found at autopsy to have pulmonary congestion and oedema, but in no instance was it possible to be sure that it was not due to aspiration.

HAEMATOLOGICAL CHANGES FOLLOWING HEAD INJURY

Any severe injury can immediately stimulate coagulation and the fibrinolytic systems. The degree of activation is said by Flute (1970) to be directly proportional to the severity of the trauma. There are now several clinical records of major coagulation changes resulting from head injuries. Goodnight et al (1974), in a prospective study of patients with acute head injury, found evidence of defibrination in nine of 13 patients in whom some destruction of brain tissue was observed at operation. Defibrination was not observed in 13 patients whose head trauma did not result in actual destruction of brain tissue. The nine patients with evidence of defibrination had haemostatic abnormalities which could well have produced intracranial bleeding, but serial testing showed a rapid return to normal within the space of a few hours. The authors of this report emphasized the need for urgent haemotological investigation whenever there was any sign of abnormal bleeding in patients with evidence of brain tissue destruction. They also suggested that it might be worth giving prophylactic treatment to patients who have suffered brain tissue damage in the hope of preventing the effects of defibrination. Vecht, Smit Sibinga and Minderhoud (1975) conducted a similar study but failed to confirm the findings of Goodnight et al (1974). They studied 34 patients with severe and moderate head injuries but found no evidence of disseminated intravascular coagulation. There was transient enhancement of fibronolytic activity, and they thought that coagulation might be activated within the first 24 hours after injury. However, their experience showed that the changes did not develop to a degree that might predispose to disseminated intravascular coagulation or to the syndrome of defibrination. We would conclude that although disseminated intravascular coagulation can occur after brain injury (Keimowitz and Annis, 1973) it is uncommon and probably does not warrant prophylactic treatment.

Anaemia can occasionally develop in the immediate postinjury period without there being any evidence of blood loss. A variety of explanations have been offered but none is entirely satisfactory. It is possible that red cell losses may result from pooling of blood, with red cell aggregation and intravascular clotting, but this is conjectural. The problem of anaemia after head injury and the possible mechanisms involved have been reviewed by McLaurin and King (1975).

REFERENCES

Altman, R. & Pruzanski, W. (1961) Post-traumatic hypopituitarism. *Annals of Internal Medicine*, **55**, 149-154.
Beckman, D. L. & Bean, J. W. (1969) Pulmonary damage and head injury. *Proceedings of the Society for Experimental Biology and Medicine*, **130**, 5-9.
Beckman, D. L., Bean, J. W. & Baslock, D. R. (1971) Sympathetic influence on lung compliance and surface forces in head injury. *Journal of Applied Physiology*, **30**, 394-399.
Binder, H. & Gerstenbrand, F. (1976) Post-traumatic vegetative syndrome. In *Handbook of Clinical Neurology.* Volume 24, *Injuries of the Brain and Skull*, Part II (Ed.) Vinken, P. J. & Bruyn, G. W. pp. 575-598. New York: American Elsevier Publishing. Amsterdam, Oxford: North Holland Publishing.
Braun, R. S. & Shoemaker, W. C. (1973) Sequential haemodynamic changes in patients with head injury: evidence for an early haemodynamic defect. *Annals of Surgery*, **177**, 187-192.
Byrne, E. A. J. (1951) Post-traumatic disturbance of hypothalamic function. *British Medical Journal*, i, 850-854.
Connor, R. C. R. (1968) Heart damage associated with intracranial lesions. *British Medical Journal,* iii, 29-31.
Croker, J. (1979) Acute gastrointestinal bleeding in the critically ill patient. *Intensive Care Medicine*, **5**, 1-4.

Crompton, M. F. (1971) Hypothalamic lesions following closed head injury. *Brain*, **94**, 165-172.

Crompton, M. F. (1975) Hypothalamic and pituitary lesions. In *Handbook of Clinical Neurology*, Volume 23, *Injuries of the Brain and Skull* Part I, (Ed.) Vinken, P. J. & Bruyn, G. W. pp. 465-470. New York: American Elsevier Publishing. Amsterdam, Oxford: North Holland Publishing.

Cushing, H. (1932) Peptic ulcers and the interbrain. *Surgery, Gynaecology & Obstetrics*, **55**, 1-33.

Daniel, P. M. & Treip, C. S. (1961) The pathology of the pituitary gland in head injury. In *Modern Trends in Endocrinology* (2nd Series). London: Butterworth.

Daniel, P. M., Pritchard, M. M. L. & Treip, C. S. (1959) Traumatic infarction of the anterior lobe of the pituitary gland. *Lancet*, **ii**, 927-931.

Dashe, A. M., Cramm, R. T., Crist, C. A., Habener, J. F. & Solomon, D. H. (1963) A water deprivation test for the differential diagnosis of polyuria. *Journal of the American Medical Association*, **185**, 699-703.

de Swiet, J. (1969) Abnormal U waves in the electrocardiogram in subarachnoid haemorrhage. *British Heart Journal*, **31**, 526-528.

Doshi, R. & Neil-Dwyer, G. (1977) Hypothalamic and myocardial lesions after subarachnoid haemorrhage. *Journal of Neurology, Neurosurgery and Psychiatry*, **40**, 821-826.

Ducker, T. B. (1968) Increased intracranial pressure and pulmonary oedema. (1) Clinical study of eleven patients. *Journal of Neurosurgery*, **38**, 112-117.

Fernando, O. U., Mariano, G. T., Gurdjian, E. S. & Hodgson, V. R. (1969) Electrocardiographic pattern in experimental concussion. *Journal of Neurosurgery*, **31**, 34-40.

Flute, P. T. (1970) Coagulation and fibrinolysis after injury. The Pathology of Trauma (Ed.) Sevitt, S. and Stoner, H. B. *Journal of Clinical Pathology*, **23** (Supplement 4), 102-109.

Golonka, J. E. & Richardson, J. A. (1970) Post-concussive hyperosmolality and deficient thirst. *American Journal of Medicine*, **48**, 261-267.

Goodnight, F. H., Kenoyer, G., Rapaport, S. I., Patch, M. J., Lee, J. A. & Kurze, T. (1974) Defibrination after brain tissue destruction. *New England Journal of Medicine*, **290**, 1043-1047.

Hersch, C. (1961) Electrocardiographic changes in head injury. *Circulation*, **23**, 853-860.

Higgins, G., Lewin, W., O'Brien, J. R. P. & Taylor, W. H. (1954) Metabolic disorders in head injury. *Lancet*, **i**, 61-67.

Hunter, J. (1772) On the digestion of the stomach after death. *Philosophical Transactions*, **B62**, 447-454.

Idjadi, F., Robbins, R., Stahl, W. M. & Essiet, G. (1971) Prospective study of gastric secretion in stressed patients with intracranial injury. *Journal of Trauma*, **11**, 681-688.

Julkunen, H., Kataja, J., Ladensuv, M. & Rokkanen, P. (1972) Electrocardiographic changes in severely injured patients treated at the intensive care unit. *Annales Chirurgiae Gynaecologiae Fenniae*, **60**, 107-111.

King, L. R., McLaurin, R. L., Lewis, H. P. & Knowles, H. C. (1970) Plasma cortisol levels after head injury. *Annals of Surgery*, **172**, 975-984.

Kornblum, R. N. & Fisher, R. F. (1969) Pituitary lesions in craniocerebral injuries. *Archives of Pathology*, **88**, 242-248.

Keimowitz, R. M. & Annis, D. L. (1973) Disseminated intravascular coagulation associated with massive brain injury. *Journal of Neurosurgery*, **39**, 178-180.

Lewin, W., Marshall, T. F., De C. & Roberts, A. H. (1979) Long term outcome after severe head injury. *British Medical Journal*, **iv**, 1533-1538.

Maroon, J. C. & Campbell, R. L. (1970) Subdural haematoma with inappropriate antidiuretic hormone secretion. *Archives of Neurology*, **22**, 234-239.

McCarthy, C. F., Wills, M. R., Keane, P. M., Gough, K. R. & Reed, A. E. (1964) The su-4855 (methopyrapone) response after head injury. *Journal of Clinical Endocrinology and Metabolism*, **24**, 121-124.

McLaurin, R. L. & King, L. R. (1975) Metabolic effects of head injury. In *Handbook of Clinical Neurology. Injuries of the Brain and Skull* Part I (Ed.) Vinken, P. J. & Bruyn, G. W. pp. 109-132. New York: American Elsevier Publishing. Amsterdam, Oxford: North Holland Publishing.

Mendelson, C. L. (1946) Aspiration of stomach contents into lungs during obstetric anaesthesia. *American Journal of Obstetrics*, **52**, 191-214.

Norton, L., Greer, J. & Eiseman, B. (1970) Gastric secretory response to head injury. *Archives of Surgery*, **101**, 200-204.

Paxson, C. L. & Brown, D. R. (1976) Post traumatic anterior hypopituitarism. *Paediatrics*, **57**, 893-896.

Payne, R. W. & De Wardener, H. E. (1958) Reversal of urinary diurnal rhythm following head injury. *Lancet*, **i**, 1098-1101.

Plum, F. & Posner, J. B. (1972) Diagnosis of stupor and coma. Edition 2. Philadelphia: F. A. Davis.

Porter, R. J. & Miller, R. A. (1948) Diabetes insipidus following closed head injury. *Journal of Neurology, Neurosurgery & Psychiatry*, **11**, 258-262.

Ross, E. J. & Christie, S. B. M. (1969) Hyponatremia. *Medicine*, **48**, 441-469.

Rudman, D., Fleischer, A. S., Kutner, M. H. & Raggio, J. F. (1977) Suprahypophyseal hypogonadism and hypothyroidism during prolonged coma after head trauma. *Journal of Clinical Endocrinology and Metabolism*, **45**, 747-754.

Simmons, R. K., Martin, A. M., Heister-Kamp, C. A. & Ducker, T. B. (1969) Respiratory insufficiency in combat casualties, 2, Pulmonary oedema following head injury. *Annals of Surgery*, **170**, 39-45.

Theodore, J. & Robin, E. D. (1975) The pathogenesis of neurogenic pulmonary oedema. *Lancet*, **ii**, 749-751.

Treip, C. S. (1970) Hypothalamic and pituitary injury. In *The Pathology of Trauma* (Ed.) Sevitt, S. & Stoner, H. B. *Journal of Clinical Pathology*, **23** (Supplement 4), 178-186.

Vecht, C. H., Smit Sibingà, C. T. & Minderhoud, J. M. (1975) Disseminated intravascular coagulation and head injury. *Journal of Neurology, Neurosurgery and Psychiatry*, **38**, 567-571.

Watts, C. C. & Clark, K. (1969) Gastric acidity in the comatose patient. *Journal of Neurosurgery*, **30**, 107-109.

Watts, C. C. & Clark, K. (1970) Effects of an anticholinergic drug on gastric acid secretion in the comatose patient. *Surgery, Gynaecology and Obstetrics*, **130**, 61-63.

Weidler, D. J. (1974) Myocardial damage and cardiac arrhythmias after intracranial haemorrhage. A critical review. *Stroke*, **5**, 368-371.

Winternitz, W. W. (1976) Pituitary failure secondary to head trauma. Case report. *Journal of Neurosurgery*, **44**, 504-505.

Witter, H. & Tascher, R. (1957) Hypophysär-hypothalamische Krankheitsbilder nach Stumpfem Schadeltrauma. *Fortschritte der Neurologie Psychiatrie*, **25**, 523-546.

Woodhall, B. (1936) Acute cerebral injuries. *Archives of Surgery*, **33**, 560-581.

Wright, P. D. (1979) Glucose homeostasis following injury. *Annals of the Royal College of Surgeons*, **61**, 427-434.

CHAPTER THIRTEEN

Management of Head Injuries

R. M. KALBAG

Trauma conventionally falls within the domain of the surgeon, but the brain offers limited scope for surgical endeavour; in treating patients with head injury the emphasis is on management, with operation playing only a minor although important role in the relief of cerebral compression and in the prevention of infection. Such a simple statement concerning the care of head injuries conceals the great divergence of opinion that exists in almost every aspect of the subject. There are manifold reasons for such divergence, and a dispassionate consideration of some of them may help to explain if not to reconcile the differences that are to be found in current neurosurgical practice.

THE DILEMMAS IN ACUTE HEAD INJURY

The emotional impact of accidental injury, the panic aroused by the sight of an unconscious and perhaps bloody casualty, the rush to obtain help: all, in varying degree, tend to blur such descriptions as may be available of what actually happened in the crucial period between injury and admission to hospital. The problem is further compounded if there is subsequent transfer to a specialist unit. Many severe injuries occur in districts that are remote from the large conurbations where major accident facilities and neurosurgical centres are situated, and often the patient's fate has been determined by the time he reaches specialist care. Frequently, neither accurate details of the accident nor information about the patient's state of consciousness soon after the injury are available. This deficiency is a matter of universal experience. Tindall and his colleagues (1975) rue the frequent oversight in obtaining a history. That they should see also the need to stress, in a paper to the 24th Annual Meeting of the Congress of Neurological Surgeons, the importance of complete examination, attention to airway, shock, level of consciousness and the possibility of multiple injury — all of which most neurosurgeons would regard as essential undergraduate knowledge — only serves to emphasize the gap between precept and practice.

Assuming that he has survived the initial hurdles, the patient if still unconscious is liable to be confronted by a surgeon, often a trainee, whose enthusiasm and possible inexperience may cloud his judgement on the appropriateness of some of the more heroic measures. In a moment of crisis, to be seen to be doing something is more comforting to anxious relatives and a more reliable safeguard against adverse comment later on than is inactivity, however masterly. There are additional incitements to activity besides the surgeon's temperament. Walker (1966) estimated that if an individual is comatose one hour after an accident, there is a 50 per cent chance that he has a mass haemorrhage with or without brain damage. Autopsy findings reported from a number of countries indicate that intracranial haemorrhage is the cause of death in about 35 to 50 per cent of fatal head injuries. If taken at their face value, Sevitt's figures (1968) alone would have important consequences on the timing and indications for radical surgery; thus 34 per cent of a series of 175 head injuries had tentorial herniation due to space-occupying lesions, mostly subdural haematomas. Such herniation often developed early and was seen in a third of those dying between one and six hours, and two-thirds of those dying during the next 18 hours. But there is no evidence that enthusiastic and aggressive surgery has done any more than perhaps make a slight dent in the mortality rates, and then at the expense of increased morbidity.

Becker et al (1977) from Richmond, Virginia, reported the results of a protocol followed over a four-year period in severe head injury. The minimum criterion for inclusion in the study was *inability to obey simple commands*.

Following assessment, endotracheal intubation and attention to breathing and circulation, each patient had a frontal twist-drill hole; after initial measurement of ventricular fluid pressure from the frontal horn, 8 ml of air were injected and portable x-ray films were taken. If there was a shift of midline structures of 5 mm or more, the patient had an immediate, extensive fronto-temporal craniotomy, which involved removal of all clot and/or necrotic brain. On the way to the operating room, the patient received intravenous Mannitol (1 g/Kg body weight). All patients, whether operated on or not, had 10 mg dexamethasone immediately and 4 mg every six hours for at least three days, were artificially ventilated and had their intracranial pressure monitored continuously. If the latter rose over 40 mm Hg (5.3 kPa), or if any increase, however small, was associated with deterioration in the level of consciousness, ventilation was increased to bring arterial $P\text{CO}_2$ down to between 20 and 25 mmHg (2.6—3.3 kPa); c.s.f. was aspirated through the ventricular catheter, or intravenous Mannitol was given. The mortality in patients so managed was 32 per cent, significantly lower than that in five other series they referred to, where the rates were between 49 per cent and 52 per cent.

All current definitions of severity of injury take into account both the degree of responsiveness at first assessment and the duration of 'coma'; when techniques like artificial ventilation are used, which make the duration of coma difficult to assess, comparisons with other types of management not involving such methods become unreliable. Decerebrate rigidity is, however, probably the least equivocal sign of severity. From Newcastle, McIver et al (1958) reported the outcome in 26 patients treated without special radiological investigation in the days before intracranial pressure monitoring or controlled ventilation were used; the emphasis was on meticulous nursing care, especially of the chest, after dealing with any surface clots revealed by exploratory burr-holes. The mortality was 38 per cent, as against 61 per cent in Becker's (1977) series of 56 comparable patients. While appreciating, not without a tinge of envy, the efficiency of the service that Becker and his colleagues have developed, one is not yet convinced of its efficacy. Jennett et al (1980) have reviewed the difficulties in establishing the value of some of the methods currently popular in the treatment of head injuries.

At the present time the pattern of care of head injuries continues, then, to be influenced by theoretical considerations of the biological properties of the brain, the experience of the surgeon, the numbers and geographical distribution of injuries, and the availability of resources, both human and financial. In this context, the following working hypotheses are necessary, especially in dealing with a head injury immediately after it has occurred:

1. The prevention or correction of anoxia from any cause is a far higher priority than the search for intracranial haematoma; a good anaesthetist has far more to offer than any surgeon.
2. The more deeply unconscious the patient, the less likely he is to benefit from dramatic surgery. In equivalent depths of coma, the patient without a haematoma has the far better prognosis.
3. The very occasional patient in desperate need of surgery can be recognized by simple criteria, as can the location of the responsible haematoma; the operative procedures required are well within the competence of any surgeon willing to carry them out.
4. The ageing brain reacts very unfavourably to injury. In the unfortunately large geriatric group, which is particularly prone to accident, surgery has little to offer.

The main priorities in the management of head injury are summarized in Table 13.1 and each item will be discussed in the following paragraphs.

Table 13.1. Priorities in head injury.

1. Prevention/correction of anoxia:
    - i. Anoxic anoxia — e.g. airway obstruction
        'flail' chest
        faciomaxillary injury
    - ii. Stagnant anoxia — due to shock ⎱ look for
    - iii. Anaemic anoxia — due to haemorrhage ⎰ injury elsewhere
2. Baseline assessment:
    - i. Level of consciousness
    - ii. External signs of injury
    - iii. Vital signs — pulse, respiration, BP, temperature
    - iv. Focal neurological deficit
3. History, especially:
    Time and circumstances of accident
    Trend in level of consciousness since injury

Anoxia

Haldane's now-famous statement that 'anoxia not only stops the machine but wrecks the machinery' was made in an article in the *British Medical Journal* in 1919. Yet one way or another hypoxia is still a frequent cause for concern among those dealing with injuries. The danger of hypoxia at its most basic level is not infrequently illustrated by the unconscious patient lying flat on his back without an airway in a casualty department or hospital bed. For such a patient, to be turned over into the 'coma' or 'recovery' position is the single initial measure that he or she requires; in the average case of concussion it is perhaps more important than any subsequent treatment that is offered. The patient should be semi-prone and almost over on to his face with his head low so that his tongue cannot fall back to obstruct his airway, while any vomit or excessive secretions in the nasopharynx can drain away with relative ease. It is the sort of attention that every layman with a rudimentary knowledge of first aid can and does give. It can be supplemented at the earliest opportunity by suction clearance of the respiratory passages and introduction of a simple airway or endotracheal tube. A wide-bore gastric tube passed through the nose, so that the stomach contents empty in to a dependent drainage bag, is an added precaution against inhalation of vomit into the lungs, especially if the trachea has not been intubated.

The importance of anoxia and the dangers of this 'second accident' cannot be emphasized too often. In my experience, the commonest cause of deteriorating consciousness is unrecognized hypoxia; it is certainly far more common than treatable acute intracranial haematoma. The usual picture is of a slow but easily recognized deterioration of consciousness occurring over the course of an hour or two. Hypoxia is not, of course, always due to neglect; it may be the consequence of commendable enthusiasm, as when an endotracheal tube is too long and goes into the right main bronchus, bypassing the left lung (Figure 13.1).

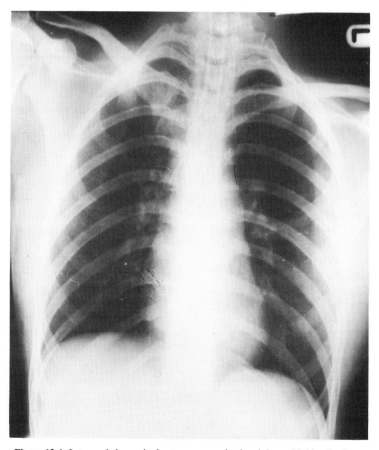

Figure 13.1. Iatrogenic hypoxia due to unrecognized endobronchial intubation.

Coma, which can arise from so many different causes besides trauma, is so common that the technique of intubation should be part of basic medical training. In Britain the experience could best be obtained during the compulsory preregistration period spent in surgery. For the vast majority undertaking this commitment who will be unlikely to take up surgery as a specialty, time spent in the anaesthetic room learning how to intubate might prove more useful in later life than that wasted hanging on to the end of an abdominal retractor.

When accidents occur at high speed there is the likelihood that injuries will be multiple; in about a quarter of such cases there is damage to the chest, with all the consequent dangers of hypoxia. The chance that such damage will go undetected is considerable. Head injury is easily recognized when a patient lies unconscious, helpless and quite possibly bleeding from the scalp, nose and ear. To look for other injuries in this circumstance calls not only for removal of layers of clothing but also for a degree of stoicism that comes only with experience. Unfortunately, by the time the young medical graduate has learned these lessons he has usually moved on into other fields where he has no opportunity to implement them. Even an obvious flail chest may be missed and pneumothorax and haemothorax are frequently overlooked.

A good working rule is that *shock means a major injury elsewhere than to the head*. Exceptions are rare enough not to matter: peripheral circulatory failure occurs as a terminal feature in severe brain damage, where cerebral compression has gone on to the stage of decompensation and where the patient is already deeply unconscious, unresponsive even to vigorous stimuli, flaccid and apnoeic. Shock may be seen rarely in adults with extensive scalp lacerations, and an infant may lose enough blood into its scalp after a closed head injury to become shocked. Shock from limb injury, such as closed fracture of the femoral shaft, demands no more than prompt transfusion; more positive action is necessary when it is due to intra-abdominal or intrathoracic haemorrhage. Most aortic ruptures after trauma are too rapidly fatal to be amenable to surgery. The same cannot be said of a ruptured spleen, lacerated viscus or avulsed kidney. We are all mindful of the tragedy of the missed extradural haematoma, but it is equally important to remember that lives may be lost as a result of treatable complications elsewhere in the body, even while patients are being transported to neurosurgical units. More frequently than is realized, lowered cerebral perfusion can produce a deterioration in consciousness to such a degree that it may mask the causative abdominal injury; the patient's inability to co-operate in the examination adds to the difficulties of diagnosis. So knowledge about the circumstances of the accident, careful noting of external signs of injury, and a high degree of suspiciousness are all of paramount importance.

Some valuable information about the influence of hypoxia on the outcome of head injury emerged from the investigation carried out by Price and Murray (1972). They studied a series of 363 survivors of head injury who had been unconscious at the time of admission to hospital. In the series they identified a hypoxic group consisting of patients with cyanosis of the lips or buccal mucosa lasting for more than ten minutes of the first 48 hours after injury, and of patients whose arterial $P\mathrm{CO_2}$ fell below 60 mm Hg (8 kPa). A hypotensive group was also identified which included patients whose blood pressure fell below the level of a —2S.D. from the mean normal systolic pressure for that patient's age and sex. The —2 S.D. level ranged from 81 mmHg (10.8 kPa) to 103 mmHg (13.7 kPa) for ages from one to 80 years, and patients were included in this group only if they were hypotensive for more than 15 minutes during their period of unconsciousness. There was also a control group consisting of patients without suggestion of even transient hypoxia or hypotension, paired by age and initial level of consciousness with patients in the other groups. From the total number, 8.5 per cent of the patients were hypoxic, 15.3 per cent were hypotensive and 3.3 per cent were both. The speed of recovery, as indicated by the periods of unconsciousness, of post-traumatic disorientation, and of time in hospital, was less in patients who were hypotensive. On the other hand, hypoxia, though it did not affect the speed of recovery, significantly reduced the chances of the patient returning to normal work. Comparing patients who were unconscious for less than one week with those who were unconscious for longer, hypoxia proved to have no significant influence in the less-severe group; but only 19 per cent of the more-severe head injuries returned to full work in comparison with 70 per cent of the control group (P<0.005). Naturally, where patients suffered both shock and cyanosis, they were even less likely to return to normal work: of the 12 patients in this category, only 7 were able to resume their original occupation, compared with all 12 of the control group (P<0.05).

Baseline Assessment

Head injury in the acute phase is a dynamic state, and it is important to establish as early as possible a baseline to which subsequent changes may be referred. If this exercise is to be of any value at all, it must be commenceable at a very early stage in the chain of events beginning at the scene of the accident; it must therefore be simple. The doctor who attacks the patient, brandishing an ophthalmoscope in one hand, and a tendon hammer in the other, is unlikely to obtain as much valuable data as the one standing by the bedside with uncluttered hands, knowing what to look for. The two most useful and perhaps sole points worth noting are the level of consciousness and the external signs of injury — the former giving a sensitive index of the degree of cerebral dysfunction, and the latter suggesting the pathological processes that may be going on inside the head.

Level of consciousness

Unconsciousness has no absolute definition, nor do terms such as stupor and coma necessarily convey the same impression to all clinicians. Coma is generally considered to be a state of unrousable unconsciousness, even to repeated noxious stimulation, yet the term comatose is regularly seen applied to patients who respond even to the extent of localizing pain. Again, stupor is usually but not invariably regarded as drowsiness from which it is difficult to rouse a patient for conversation at a simple level; but there is at least one respectable monograph on head injury which refers to a patient as being stuporose despite a purposeful and vigorous response to painful stimulation. Even our illustrious literary forebear, the great Dr Peter Mark Roget, considered coma and stupor to be synonymous.

Apart from these terminological difficulties, considerable confusion also arises from the various methods that have been advocated for grading the depth of coma. The level of consciousness can most clearly be described in terms of the best response to a series of increasingly powerful stimuli, including the nature and speed of that response. Simplicity is important in any common urgent problem, but to divide levels of consciousness into watertight categories is to impose an unrealistic rigidity on what, in fact, is a continuous spectrum.

On approaching an injured person, the logical first step is to note his reaction to the spoken word. Is he alert? Can he give his name, age and address? Does he know where he is, what time of the day or day of the week it is? Are his answers appropriate to the questions asked? Can one understand at all what he is saying? In the absence of a verbal response, will he carry out simple requests? If not, does he resent interference of a simple type, such as attempts to take his pulse, look into his eyes or undress him? If there is still no response, more potent painful stimuli are used; the patient may localize the pain to ward it off. At deeper levels of unconsciousness, the response may be non-specific, decorticate or decerebrate. Finally, there may be no response at all to the most vigorous stimulation, except, perhaps, a change in respiratory rhythm.

Teasdale and Jennett (1974) have evolved a 'coma scale' (see Table 6.3, p. 45) which comes closer than anything previously described to providing a relatively unambiguous form of recording. It depends upon three categories of behavioural response — eye-opening, verbal and motor reactions, each being divided into distinct hierarchical grades. To the writer, the most attractive feature of the Glasgow Coma Scale is its departure from the traditional emphasis on changes in pupillary size and the quality of the light reflex as an indication of the possible need for surgical intervention. To wait until a pupil has dilated and the light reflex has been abolished is to delay action until the integrity of the midbrain has become seriously threatened. In most cases, a decision to operate would have been made earlier by noting deterioration in consciousness alone. On rare occasions, when a patient is deeply unconscious from the time of injury and totally unresponsive, pupillary inequality may be the only obvious change; in my experience, surgery in such a patient has not improved the gloomy outlook in any way.

External signs of injury

The location of an acute intracranial haematoma can be more confidently related to the point of external impact than to localizing neurological signs, however carefully elicited. Recording of the external signs of injury is therefore a very important part of the baseline assessment.

In less urgent circumstances, ecchymotic discolouration of the taut skin over the mastoid process — Battle's sign — may mean a fracture of the petrous temporal bone; this, together with bleeding from the ear on that side, demands prophylactic antibiotics for a compound fracture of the floor of the middle fossa, especially when a patient's restlessness may not allow confirmation of the lesion by x-rays of adequate quality. A subconjunctival haemorrhage stopping at the sclerocorneal junction accompanied by bleeding from the nose are useful pointers to a possible compound fracture of the anterior cranial fossa. A bruise near the outer edge of the eyebrow with a dilated pupil on that side suggest that the pupillary dilatation may be due to an optic nerve injury.

Vital signs

In the acute stage, the pulse, blood pressure and respiration are more important as an alert to the medical attendants of a possible systemic injury elsewhere, than as an indication of the presence of a rapidly expanding intracranial mass lesion. A slowing of the pulse and a high blood pressure are, indeed, well-recognized signs of rising intracranial pressure, but it is less well known that this — the Cushing response — is neither a constant nor an early phenomenon in intracranial hypertension. Nevertheless, as ancillary signs of cerebral dysfunction, they have a definite place in management.

Neurological examination

Only examination of the simplest sort is required in the acute phase of injury, over and above that which relates to the determination of the level of consciousness. Ocular movements, pupil size and reaction, limb weakness, abnormalities of muscle tone and plantar responses: these are the few main points that need to be noted. Further elaboration will depend on the attitude and interest of the examiner, and may be out of place in the atmosphere of the average busy accident department. The emphasis is on signs that, when they begin to change, signify deterioration in the neurological state, although it is quite exceptional for such changes to occur without a simultaneous deepening of coma. These signs, especially the development of pupillary inequality, may become important where changes in ward staff incur the risk of missing minor, but significant, alterations in the level of consciousness. Again, plantar responses that change from flexor to extensor are more easily appreciated than subtle changes in limb weakness. The development of neck stiffness has sometimes been a useful index in management. If there is no associated Kernig's sign, the neck rigidity may be due to tonsillar herniation through the foramen magnum: if there is a positive Kernig's sign, the patient may have meningitis. If meningism is present from the outset, it is likely that there has been a traumatic subarachnoid haemorrhage; the blood may have come from a lacerated cortex, in which case the prospects of a subdural haematoma forming are heightened significantly.

History

Contrary to usual clinical practice, it is best to leave the history-taking till the patient has been resuscitated and a baseline examination completed. The importance of history in the management of head injury is insufficiently appreciated, and the necessary information is, more often than not, wanting. Most important is the trend in consciousness since the accident — is the casualty improving, unchanged or deteriorating, and, if the last, in what way? The circumstances of the accident can help anticipate the pattern of injury and the possibility of other organs being involved. The time at which the accident occurred, together with the changing pattern of consciousness, serve as valuable guides to the speed of evolution of the clinical state and help to indicate if there is time for ancillary investigation, or if immediate surgery is imperative.

THE ADMISSION OF HEAD INJURIES TO HOSPITAL

Head injuries impose a considerable burden on accident departments. In a large central city hospital in Glasgow, Scotland, they account for 20 per cent of all acute surgical admissions, but two-thirds of them are fully conscious without neurological symptoms or signs and without skull fracture (Galbraith, 1973). The decision to admit a head injury to hospital (Table 13.2) is dictated largely by conventional attitudes, some of which are questionable.

A patient who arrives in hospital unconscious or with symptoms of cerebral dysfunction is an obvious candidate for admission. Unfortunately, the restless, confused and sometimes violent drunk falls into this category, and he may be very hard to distinguish from the much rarer head-injured patient with traumatic subarachnoid

Table 13.2.   Criteria for admission to hospital.

1.	Obvious signs/symptoms of cerebral disturbance — unconsciousness, confusion, drowsiness, headache, vomiting, fits, focal neurological deficit.
2.	Imperative asymptomatic patients with compound/depressed skull fracture.
3.	Arguable asymptomatic patients with a. history of unconsciousness b. simple linear fracture.

haemorrhage or in the early phase of evolution of an intracranial haematoma. Increasing restlessness is an unusual but well-known presentation of an extradural haematoma. Therefore the drunks have to be catered for. However, their admission to an ordinary surgical ward can create disturbances that are beyond the imagination of those who have not had the experience of looking after them. Invariably these inebriates arrive by night and disturb the sleep of other patients. Nursing staff is often at its lowest level at this time, and the increased demand on nursing time required merely to control a restless patient without sedation can detract from the vital care that ill patients may require. A short-stay ward, near the casualty department and set aside for those patients who need no more than overnight observation, is a reasonable and necessary compromise, not always provided in hospitals.

There are patients whose admission may be imperative, but who have never lost consciousness and are completely symptom-free when first seen in hospital, usually because of a scalp laceration. It is in this group that errors in management often occur. *Every patient seen in the casualty department who does not warrant admission on clinical grounds should have his skull x-rayed if there is any sign or history of injury about the head or face.* The radiological demonstration of a fracture in such a patient should normally be an indication for taking him into hospital. Failure to appreciate the presence of a fracture underneath an apparently simple scalp laceration can result in a fatal meningitis or cerebral abscess.

In this country the recommended practice is to admit to hospital for observation all patients with a skull fracture, however simple it may appear to be radiologically. The belief is that this will keep to a minimum the disastrously high mortality from extradural haematoma. It can be argued that, in fact, complications in this group develop so infrequently that the level of surveillance by over-worked night nurses is likely to be no higher than that which a watchful and well-briefed relative can provide at home. The fact remains that three-quarters of all patients who develop an extradural haematoma have a fracture, and careful observation in hospital of all patients with skull fracture is the ideal to aim at in the early detection of this rare, but eminently treatable, complication of head injury.

The position in children may be different. Harwood-Nash, Hendrick and Hudson (1971) studied 1187 children with skull fractures, who constituted 26.6 per cent of 4465 consecutive admissions with head injury to the Toronto Hospital for Sick Children. They concluded that the presence of a skull fracture alone, without associated clinical evidence of damage to the central nervous system, is of little significance; it should not alter decisions about management, except when the fracture is compound or depressed. In this series, fractures were seen in less than half of the children who had extradural haematomas, whilst subdural haematoma was twice as common in children without fracture as it was in those with fracture.

The series would suggest that there is little point in admitting an asymptomatic child merely because of a simple fracture, provided that there is a responsible person at home who can be relied upon to bring the patient back to hospital if symptoms such as headache, confusion or repeated vomiting develop. This is certainly a consideration of some importance in children, where the very real hazard of psychological trauma due to hospital admission has to be weighted against the theoretical advantage of a period under observation.

The other debatable group conventionally observed in hospital comprises those patients who have been concussed but, when seen in the casualty department, are alert, rational and symptom-free and whose skull x-rays show no fracture. If admission of such patients is arranged because of the risk of the development of an extradural haematoma, the point should be made that the latter is more consistently related to the presence of skull fracture than to a history of concussion. An extradural haematoma is a complication of skull injury rather than of brain injury; concussion is a sign of the latter. The admission of patients in the category under consideration is influenced by anecdotes told about individuals sent home from casualty departments because they were conscious, but who later developed fatal or near-fatal complications. On the rare occasions when the writer has met this situation, closer enquiry has invariably shown that, though the patient was talking and able to give his name and address, he was either confused or showing some evidence of cerebral dysfunction that was mistaken for drunkenness; such a patient does not come into the category under discussion. There is, however, another possible indication for the admission of these patients. It is that gradual mobilization and rehabilitation after even minor concussion may help to overcome postconcussional syndromes. If this is the intention then overnight stay with peremptory discharge and no follow-up, as is the custom, is illogical, especially as a significant number of patients develop postural vertigo. Cairns (1941) suggested that a head-injured person with a post-traumatic amnesia of five minutes to one hour is not fit to return to full work for at least four to six weeks. Relander, Troupp and Bjorkesten (1972) found that active rehabilitation of patients after relatively minor head injury reduced the average time off work to 18 days, as compared with 32 days in those merely discharged with reassurance. But since the enthusiasm and the resources for such rehabilitation are generally wanting, the admission of this group of patients panders to blind ritual rather than to reasoned practice.

A reassessment of the indications for the admission of minor head injuries into hospital would do more than conserve scarce resources. The average surgical or accident ward has to cope with so many head injuries requiring no specific surgical treatment that it may lose sight of the purpose of such admission, and the very occasional patient who needs urgent operation may not be recognized in time. If brief inquiry in an asymptomatic patient shows that he is not being sent away to spend the night on his own, and if, as an added precaution, the patient's relative is provided with a card bearing simple details of warning symptoms, it would seem reasonable not to detain him. Until a rational approach to the management of head injury becomes more widely accepted, one's advice to the junior medical practitioner, who often has to make a decision without reference to his seniors, would be to admit when in doubt.

Skull X-rays in the Casualty Department

Theoretically, skull x-rays taken at an early stage in the management of a head injury should be of value in anticipating complications, so they should be obtained as soon as possible after resuscitation and initial assessment. This is another area in which precept takes little account of the problems encountered in practice. Most head injuries come in by night when hospital staffing is at its lowest ebb, and where a radiographer either has to be fetched from home or is the only one on duty and busy with other emergencies. Delays of an hour or more, during which the patient is hanging around the hospital corridors, are the rule rather than the exception. Deterioration may be missed and undoubtedly on odd occasions a patient may die on the x-ray table, either from aspirating vomit into the lungs or from respiratory arrest due to an unrecognized extradural clot. Routine x-ray during the night is thus not without hazard. And even in cases where no harm does in fact come to him, the patient is often restless and confused, so that the radiographs are of little value and have to be repeated at a later stage when he is more co-operative. If an acute intracranial haematoma develops, it is more reliably localized by reference to the circumstances of the accident and the point of impact on the head than on the basis of demonstrable skull fractures.

The following points are suggested guidelines for skull radiography in the casualty department:

1. If the decision to admit a patient has already been made on clinical grounds, defer skull x-rays until the following day.
2. Where the patient is deteriorating rapidly and an intracranial haematoma has already been diagnosed, do not waste precious time taking skull x-rays.
3. If the suspicion of multiple trauma, especially to the chest, spine or abdomen, makes x-rays necessary, a doctor must stay by the patient throughout the procedure.
4. X-rays must be taken before sending home a patient who does not qualify for admission on clinical grounds.

INDICATIONS FOR SURGERY

Out of the thousands of patients with head injury admitted to hospital, only a few need surgical treatment beyond the simple suture of scalp lacerations. Further indications can be considered in three categories, in order of decreasing urgency:

1. Relief of cerebral compression.
2. Prevention of intracranial infection.
3. Correction of cosmetic handicaps.

Rare conditions such as caroticocavernous fistula may call for surgical intervention, but it is very doubtful if operations for intractable post-traumatic epilepsy or persistent dyskinesia have any place at all.

That cerebral compression should be dealt with as soon as it is recognized is a fundamental and undisputed principle, although how it should be done and what result may be considered acceptable are matters for debate. Compound fractures of the vault of the skull, especially if depressed, need to be treated with the same respect as compound ones anywhere else in the body; their management is essentially along the lines indicated in the first chapter or two of all good undergraduate textbooks of surgery.

Repair of a compound fracture at the base of the skull is best postponed to a stage when the operation may be considered an 'elective' or planned procedure and not an emergency. Cosmetic operations would include the delayed repair of skull defects left after operations for the hurried evacuation of acute intracranial haematomas or after contaminated comminuted fractures. Most surgeons would also regard the elevation of a simple depressed fracture as no more than a cosmetic operation. Some of these points will be considered in greater detail at a later stage in the chapter.

INTRACRANIAL HAEMATOMA

Mortality and morbidity in acute head injury remain high, despite the application of increasingly sophisticated diagnostic methods and intensive therapeutic regimes. Delays in diagnosis and treatment can be corrected by better organization and improved training of medical and nursing staff in the recognition of minor changes in the level of consciousness. But better roads and faster cars have overtaken the efforts of the medical profession, so much so that Jamieson (1970), in reviewing his own experience of subdural haematomas, wondered 'Is our vision wide enough to look beyond our parochial technical problems, and our humanity great enough to take up the challenges and responsibilities involved in accident prevention?'

Clinical diagnosis of haematoma (Table 13.3)

A progressive deterioration in the level of consciousness is the most reliable index of rising intracranial pressure, whether due to surface haematoma or to brain swelling. The importance of careful serial recording of levels of consciousness has already been emphasized.

Table 13.3. Acute surface haematoma after head injury: differential diagnosis.

Clinical features: deteriorating consciousness
increasing focal neurological deficit
increasing restlessness.

	Extradural	Subdural
Incidence	Rare	Relatively common
Age	Mostly under 20	Any age but especially extremes of life
Type of accident	Often trivial	High speed Severe impact
Direction of injury	Lateral	Anteroposterior usually back of head
Site of haematoma	Under point of impact	Low frontotemporal
Prognosis	Excellent with prompt surgery	Often bad despite heroic efforts

N.B. There are always exceptions. Both may occur in a single patient. Both may be difficult to distinguish from brain swelling.

Restlessness in a patient after head injury is generally due to a full bladder, but *increasing restlessness* is a more ominous though rare sign of slowly evolving surface haematoma, usually extradural; it is often accompanied by the persistent rubbing of a particular area of the scalp, which virtually tells the surgeon the position of the clot. The significance of pupillary change and increasing hemiparesis has been alluded to previously, and these are particularly relevant when levels of consciousness have not been diligently noted. The vital signs — pulse, respiration and blood pressure — are perhaps more important in multiple injuries than in pure head injuries for identifying unrecognized extracranial complications that have produced alterations in consciousness through subclinical hypoxia.

If a surface haematoma is suspected, it can be localized in most cases by considering three factors: the patient's age, the nature of the accident and the point of external impact. The principles of clinical localization are better understood if one looks at some of the basic facts behind each of the two most frequently diagnosed lesions — extradural and subdural haematoma.

Extradural Haematoma

An extradural haematoma is an acute and eminently treatable complication of blunt head injury; it is relatively rare and is seen in less than 0.5 per cent of head injuries admitted to hospital. In communities where the car does not figure prominently in the causation of accidents, where high road speeds cannot be attained and where arguments are settled with sticks and stones rather than with fists, knives or guns, the lesion is more common.

The haematoma is more accurately labelled as extradural than as 'middle meningeal', because bleeding is not necessarily from middle meningeal vessels; indeed it is not invariably arterial, as is generally supposed. All standard textbooks of anatomy mention that the vascular marking on the inner table of the skull is due to the middle meningeal vein, and that the artery lies outside the bone. This point was forcefully brought out by Wood Jones (1912). Veins have thin walls and, unlike arteries, they can rupture easily. This accounts for the fact that relatively trivial blows, especially to the side of the head, can precipitate extradural haemorrhage. Nearly 30 per cent of patients with this potentially lethal complication have had nonconcussional head injuries, often too slight to have taken them to a doctor in the first instance (Gallagher and Browder, 1968).

With advancing years, the dura becomes increasingly adherent to the skull and difficult to separate from the inner table. This is why extradural haematoma is essentially an affliction of youth. More than half of those affected are under the age of 20, and it is a rare condition over 40. It is, however, exceptional in infancy, when a blow tends to indent the pliable skull and dura together so that any damage inflicted is directly borne by the brain, and haematoma collects more often inside the dura mater than outside.

Every review article on the subject of extradural haematoma makes reference to Sir Charles Bell's observation of 1816 that, when the cadaveric cranium was struck with a wooden mallet, the blow caused the dura to become separated from the skull directly beneath the site of impact. This, of course, is where the clot invariably forms.

Prognosis is determined by two factors: the severity of the primary brain damage and the extent to which the secondary disturbance due to distortion of the brain stem has progressed before surgery can be undertaken. Despite what has been said in previous paragraphs, extradural haematomas are occasionally seen after severe injury, but in this circumstance their evacuation does not alter the outcome. An extreme example in the writer's experience was of a patient suffering an extradural haemorrhage after a motorcycle accident; both internal carotid arteries in the cavernous sinuses had been transected by a fracture of the base of the skull through the pituitary fossa, and survival time was less than half an hour from the moment of impact. In practice, if a patient has been deeply unconscious and unresponsive from the beginning, he is not going to be helped by surgery. If a patient who was reacting briskly and localizing light stimuli on admission has been allowed to deteriorate to a stage where his pupils are widely dilated and he is apnoeic, then death, or at best a persistent vegetative state, is virtually certain. In 1772, an extradural haematoma was successfully treated by a Mr J. Hill in Dumfries in Scotland (Gallagher and Browder, 1968), so when congratulating ourselves on the great strides made in British surgery we should pause to consider that, 200 years later, patients still occasionally die while being transferred to a distant neurological department from a district general hospital.

Subdural haematoma

Unlike the extradural haematoma, the subdural form is an all-too-common complication of head injury, with a mortality and morbidity far higher than might be judged from most surgical textbooks. It is most likely to occur after high speed injury, where the direction of the force is anteroposterior and the point of impact is at the back of the head. Bleeding occurs from lacerations of the tip of the temporal lobe and the undersurface of the frontal lobes, caused by the edges of the lesser wings of the sphenoid, either on both sides or on the side opposite to the point of impact on the skull. In infants or in cases where there is an associated fracture, depressed or otherwise, the cortex directly under the point of impact may be lacerated. Exceptionally, an elderly patient with marked cerebral atrophy may develop an acute subdural collection of blood from a torn superior cerebral vein without any associated cerebral laceration.

The prognosis after an acute subdural haematoma is governed more by the severity of the original impact and the rapidity with which the bleeding has occurred than by the speed and skill with which measures are applied to deal with it. In this respect it differs from the chronic subdural haematoma, which is an almost totally different entity.

The following classification of subdural haematoma, adapted from Hooper (1969), is of practical value as a guide in management.

1. The 'explosive' or rapidly fatal extravasation — usually from a violent impact. The patient is deeply unconscious from the outset and soon the classical signs of compression develop; there is decerebrate rigidity, pupillary dilatation and inequality. Death ensues within six to 12 hours, regardless of treatment.

2. Acute subdural haematoma — the pattern evolves rather more slowly within the first 24 hours; at least, it is slow enough to permit recognition of an early period of recovery, however slight, before deterioration sets in. Mortality in this group is about 75 per cent, despite energetic treatment. Good recovery is rare and occurs mostly in those under the age of 20. The cases with the most favourable outcome include those patients who were almost able to talk shortly after injury. Conventionally all haematomas presenting within the first 72 hours are considered acute but, in my experience, those coming to operation after 24 hours have a mortality approximately equal to that in the subacute group. In these patients, craniotomy is less likely to be disappointing than in the acute cases, where an extensive operation achieves no more than does a limited craniectomy.

3. Subacute subdural haematoma — this group consists mostly of patients whose progress after injury has not been entirely satisfactory, with recovery being slow or incomplete so that discharge from hospital is delayed. Notable deterioration may occur from the second day onwards, and usually begins within three weeks of the injury. Mortality is less than 20 per cent; those most at risk are the ones in whom the haematoma develops early. However, this group carries significant morbidity in terms of neurological deficit and post-traumatic epilepsy.

4. The 'fleeting' subdural haematoma — when computerized tomography is used routinely in the assessment of head injuries then occasional subdural collections, up to one centimetre in depth, may be demonstrated in patients who appeared clinically to

have no such complication. If operation is deferred, these collections may resolve spontaneously. In some neurosurgical services it has been the practice to make routine burr holes in all patients who are still unconscious on admission to hospital, and in this circumstance surgery will take undue credit for the cure of a small number of subdural haematomas which would have recovered in any event.

5. The chronic subdural haematoma — this is characteristically seen in the middle-aged and elderly. A history of head injury, obtained even in retrospect, is the exception rather than the rule, and patients with this condition are generally seen in medical departments. The usual picture is of a patient past the age of 50 years with fluctuating confusion and drowsiness, bilateral ptosis, small pupils, a defect of conjugate-upward gaze, neck stiffness, brisk tendon reflexes without marked weakness of the limbs, but with bilateral extensor plantar responses. Unlike the acute haematomas, the chronic forms tend to be high on the convexity of the cerebral hemisphere; they are generally fluid and may be treated simply by making burr holes. The prognosis is usually excellent.

Whilst they are not strictly haematomas, collections of xanthochromic fluid under tension may sometimes be found incidentally when the former are being sought. They are referred to as subdural hygromas and their aetiology is uncertain. The acute hygroma is to some extent analagous to the tension pneumothorax, with a valvular tear in the arachnoid preventing re-entry of cerebrospinal fluid into the subarachnoid space. Sometimes the patient can be obviously improved just by making a burr hole, even though no particular steps have been taken to deal with the presumed one-way valve.

Investigation of Suspected Haematoma

The modern neurosurgeon has at his disposal a fine array of diagnostic aids, but special investigation will not in the foreseeable future entirely supplant clinical judgement in cases of suspected haematoma. Not all patients suffer their injuries in the neighbourhood of neurosurgical units and patients with extradural haematomas may not survive until special investigations are completed. Jamieson and Yelland (1968), discussing the results of their own very large series of extradural haematomas, wrote as follows: 'The neurosurgeon who from within his ivory tower writes of the necessity for or the desirability of special investigation, radiological or otherwise, instead of emphasising simple clinical appraisal, or who advocates osteoplastic flap craniotomy, does a grave disservice to the injured. Not only does he jeopardise the chances of that large number of patients who cannot benefit directly from his own care, but he is also likely to find that his own mortality rate, based on such a policy, is higher than that desirable or attainable'.

As a working rule, all patients with closed head injuries in whom there is a suspicion of intracranial haematoma within six hours after injury should be operated upon, without recourse to special investigation, if any of the following conditions prevail:

1. The patient is unconscious but is known to have spoken after the injury.
2. The level of consciousness is deteriorating noticeably even in the course of initial examination.
3. The patient has become decerebrate in hospital when he was not so before admission.
4. The patient is decerebrate and no history is available.

Burr hole exploration

This chapter is not intended to be a manual for surgeons; but it may not be out of place to include a brief discussion of surgical principle under this heading, in an attempt to dispel some of the anxiety and mystery that surround the whole subject of acute head injury. Even though acute intracranial haematomas are of relatively infrequent occurrence, as already discussed, the burr hole should still be regarded as the diagnostic tool most readily available to the surgeon in cases of doubt. As his experience increases, the surgeon will find that he makes fewer negative burr holes, but even a specialist unit should expect to include in its figures a small number of negative explorations. (If this is not the case, perhaps it is becoming less vigilant than it should be, and the speed with which its theatre facilities can be mobilized in an emergency may be found to have declined.) Exploration rarely requires more than three burr holes. The first is placed at the site where an extradural haematoma is most likely to be, namely at the point of impact; it may be seen more clearly when the head is shaved and it may appear as a bruise, a 'bogginess' of the scalp or a laceration, especially if it is at the side or the front of the head. If there is no blood clot at this site, either outside or underneath the dura, a second burr hole should be made low in the anterior temporal region on the opposite side, to look for a possible subdural collection. A third, if necessary, should be made on the side of the injury in the temporal region, again searching for a subdural collection. When the point of impact is occipital, temporal burr holes alone are probably all that is required, as it is unlikely that there will be an extradural haematoma.

After the first clot encountered has been dealt with, preferably by a craniectomy, in which the initial burr hole is enlarged with bone rongeurs, possible clots on the opposite side should still be ruled out. This is not, however, necessary if there has been a clear-cut lucid interval after the injury, or if after evacuation of the first clot the pressure within the dura is low, provided of course that no additional methods of reducing intracranial tension have been employed.

Once a burr hole has located an extradural haematoma, the situation is no longer critical and the next step will depend on the surgeon's confidence in his own ability to complete the operation. He must resist the temptation to suck out the clot before he has room to deal with the bleeding. As the burr hole is made, the soft dark clot extrudes spontaneously and thus gradually relieves the intracranial pressure, whilst at the same time sufficient clot remains behind to prevent fierce bleeding from torn dural vessels. A patient in this situation can travel safely, by ordinary ambulance if necessary, to a neurosurgical unit with his wound left open; the head should be lightly swathed in dressings to soak up any bleeding which, as a rule, is surprisingly scanty.

'Head injuries travel well' is a statement that has often been quoted since it first appeared in a War Surgery Supplement. In statistical terms the statement is probably true, because urgent operation rarely affects the prognosis for head injuries except in the case of extradural haematoma, and this particular lesion is not encountered often enough to make any appreciable impact on overall mortality.

The 'three burr hole method' will locate the vast majority of intracranial clots, but not all of them. If there is any anxiety that an atypical clot may have been missed, a further burr hole should be made; preference is for a right frontal hole 2.5 cm from the midline and near the coronal suture, to needle the lateral ventricle. If the ventricle is easily entered and large amounts of cerebrospinal fluid are obtained, it may be that there is a haematoma in the posterior fossa, though this is rare. If the lateral ventricle is very small or if it is displaced and difficult to find, there are two further sites that can be explored. If the patient has a black eye, indicative of an anterior fossa fracture, the burr hole may be placed low in the forehead just above the eye; alternatively, and particularly if there is discolouration over the mastoid process, it is worth making a burr hole in the posterior temporal area, again low down.

Echoencephalography

Echoencephalography is a safe bedside technique, and at first glance a very attractive screening test for use in the casualty department. But a reliable midline echo can only be obtained after very considerable practice and, without this, the investigation may be misleading. Thomson and Longley (1965, personal communication) reviewed 1445 echograms carried out on patients in whom the position of the midline structures was independently identified by means of straight x-rays showing a calcified pineal, by angiograms showing the internal verebral vein, or by ventriculograms demonstrating the position of the third ventricle. They showed that the echogram was less reliable in patients with intracranial pathology than in those who were normal. There was a 9.2 per cent error in recognizing displacement of midline structures and, even though this error was smaller than in many published series, it was felt that the investigation was scarcely adequate for the discrimination required of it.

Nevertheless, echoencephalography does have a useful, although limited, role in a number of situations:

1. When a patient with multiple injuries needs sedation, for example in the case of of controlled ventilation for a flail chest, ordinary observation may not be feasible, and serial echograms may help to identify the development of intracranial haematoma.
2. If a patient has had an angiogram which is either normal or shows a haematoma or contusion which is to be treated expectantly, repeated echograms may provide a simple and relatively satisfactory method of monitoring progress.

Carotid angiography and computerized axial tomography

Cerebral angiography has been the definitive diagnostic procedure in the management of head injuries for many years, but it has now been superseded by computerized axial tomography — the 'CT scan'. In addition to being noninvasive, the scan gives more information about precise pathology and it can differentiate between haematoma, oedema and infarction, which the angiogram is unable to do. But in spite of the considerable diagnostic benefits of the scan, its overall contribution in the management of head injuries must inevitably be limited because of the logistical problems in their management. Thus in 1972 in England and Wales there were 5175 deaths from head injury; 40 per cent of the deaths occurred before patients reached hospital and 20 per cent of the total died in hospital before they could actually be admitted.

In a perplexing situation, if time and facilities permit, the surgeon will be more reassured by a normal scan than by negative burr holes, which can leave lingering doubts about missed pathology. Furthermore, where pathology does exist, definitive special investigations may provide precise knowledge about its nature and location, which will allow the surgeon to plan his approach and limit the extent of his operation to a minimum. He may be able to achieve what he requires through a craniotomy, whereas without special investigation he might have to resort to craniectomy, with the additional problem of a skull defect which will have to be repaired at a later date. But angiography and, even more so, the CT scan create problems of their own. They reveal lesions that were not suspected clinically, and these may pose problems in management. Thus, temporal lobe contusion became an increasingly frequent diagnosis as the popularity of angiography grew and it was sometimes a difficult decision whether or not excision should be carried out. In fact, surgery is seldom required and certainly the decision should be made on clinical rather than on radiological grounds.

French and Dublin (1977) evaluated the role of computerized tomography in a thousand consecutive head injuries; 161 out of 316 patients who were scanned had abnormalities, in 38 per cent more than one, yet only 91 needed any operation. Equally interesting was the finding that 13 per cent of alert asymptomatic patients had abnormal scans, while six patients with an initially normal investigation developed complications later. A negative investigation soon after injury does not absolve attendants of the responsibility of continuing vigilance.

The influence of the CT scan on the management of head injuries was also studied by Ambrose, Gooding and Uttley (1976). Three groups, each consisting of 100 consecutive patients with head injury transferred to a busy neurosurgical department, were analysed retrospectively. Group I consisted of patients who were admitted during the period before the CT scan was available. Group II were patients who were treated immediately after the technique was established, and Group III were patients who were referred at a time when the scan was firmly established as a method of investigation. A comparison between Groups I and III was instructive, and the following points emerged:

1. Group III had at least one CT scan, and there was a dramatic fall in the number of other investigations performed, from 61 to 16.
2. The number of exploratory operations fell from 33 to two.
3. There was no change in the overall mortality.

The study thus confirmed the theoretical expectation that computerized tomography would reduce the morbidity from invasive investigations and from exploratory surgery, without influencing the overall mortality. The most obvious indication for computerized tomography or angiography is a progressive deterioration in the neurological state that is not dramatic enough to threaten life immediately. Another circumstance in which such investigation is important is where the history is uncertain and the patient remains unconscious for no obvious reason. Likewise, scanning is particularly useful in patients whose management, for one reason or another, involves techniques that interfere with the normal assessment procedures. It is important to reiterate the previous caveat that one normal investigation is no guarantee against later complication, and serial scanning may sometimes be called for.

In CT scanning, fresh blood is seen as a dense white image, biconvex if extradural (Figure 13.2), and diffuse concavo-convex if subdural (Figure 13.3). Oedema shows up as less dense than normal brain, while contusions have a mottled appearance. At operation, an acute subdural haematoma may be much thicker than the scan suggests. The density of a clot generally decreases with age, and may sometimes be isodense with adjacent brain; such a clot may not be recognized, other than as a displacement of the midline structures, and may be missed altogether if bilateral haematomas prevent any such displacement. A chronic subdural haematoma is less dense than brain and, if wholly fluid, its ouline is biconvex.

Angiography may still be indicated when scans are equivocal, or in suspected vascular lesions such as traumatic carotid thrombosis or caroticocavernous fistula.

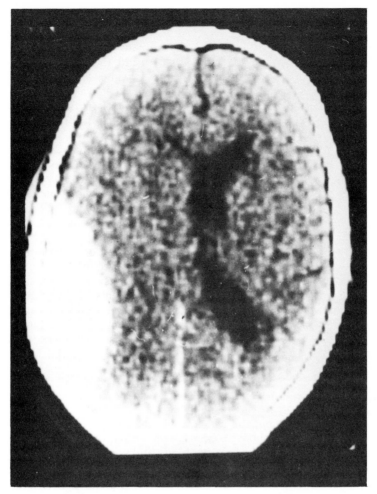

Figure 13.2. CT scan showing acute extradural haematoma.

Other investigations

Ventriculography. This involves the introduction of a positive or negative contrast medium into the lateral ventricles through a burr hole, prior to radiological examination. Where intracranial pressure is already high the procedure may make the patient much worse, and it has therefore never found favour in the management of acute head injuries. One possible exception occurs where exploratory burr holes have shown a tense brain but no surface clot; in this circumstance it may be more expedient to cannulate the ventricle and reduce the pressure, whilst at the same time introducing air or oxygen, than to delay whilst organizing an angiogram or CT scan.

Lumbar puncture. This technique has no place in the diagnosis or management of most head injuries. Indeed, if it is carried out indiscriminately in patients whose intracranial pressure is raised, it may have fatal results. It is, of course, necessary when meningitis is suspected, as for instance when there is fever and neck stiffness. It is,

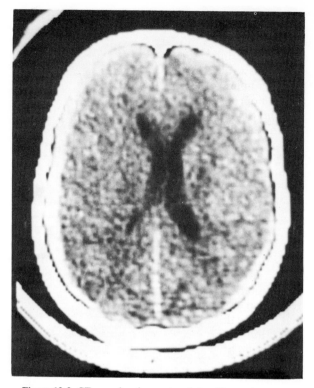

Figure 13.3. CT scan showing acute subdural haematoma.

however, important to rule out the presence of a haematoma in the first instance. In cases of traumatic subarachnoid haemorrhage, lumbar draining of blood-stained cerebrospinal fluid may help to reduce morbidity and prevent the later development of hydrocephalus.

Lumbar air encephalography. This has all the disadvantages of lumbar puncture and is not used in the management of acute head injuries. It is, however, sometimes of value in the chronic situation where occult hydrocephalus is suspected.

Radioisotope cisternography. The technique is recommended for the diagnosis of communicating hydrocephalus. It has the advantage that it is a dynamic study which enables the passage of c.s.f. and isotope between the ventricles and the subarachnoid space to be followed by serial examination. For the patient, it is less disturbing than an air encephalogram, but the early claims that were made for the reliability of this investigation have not quite come up to expectation.

Radioisotope encephalography. The method has been largely superseded by the CT scan, although it is still of some value in centres where the latter is not available; it sometimes obviates the need to carry out angiography in elderly or arteriopathic patients.

The electroencephalogram. This is used in some intensive care units for the diagnosis of irreversible brain death, but there are many who would not regard it as essential for this purpose. It does not have a significant part to play in the management of acute head injury.

Operative Procedures

The procedure for dealing with a haematoma that has been found on burr hole exploration or after special investigation is governed by two factors: the rate of deterioration of the patient's condition and the experience of the surgeon concerned. As a general rule, where burr holes have been made because of the urgency of the situation, a craniectomy is most appropriate. In a craniectomy, the original scalp incision is extended and the burr hole enlarged by nibbling away bone until there is a large enough opening to deal with the clot. This is a particularly suitable approach in the management of acute extradural haematoma, where the clot gradually squeezes itself out while access is being obtained; it is a procedure that any surgeon can cope with. There is a common misconception that burr hole evacuation of fluid blood is sufficient in the very acute subdural haematoma. The only intradural clot that can be treated successfully with such a simple procedure is the fleeting subdural, which does not need surgery anyway. Any collection of blood that has accumulated rapidly enough to threaten life must have come from a torn vessel or vessels, whose bleeding cannot be stopped through a burr hole. The least that is required in these circumstances is a subtemporal craniectomy to deal with bleeding cortical vessels and to excise part of the inevitably damaged and swollen temporal lobe. Where it has been possible to carry out angiography and computerized tomography in advance, a craniotomy to provide adequate exposure and to control bleeding then becomes feasible, using pressure-control methods that remove the urgency from the operation.

The preceding section is an outline of the author's policy in all patients coming to surgery more than 24 hours after injury. When operation becomes imperative earlier, for instance because of an intradural lesion, craniectomy is generally carried out, provided that the patient is sufficiently conscious to show, at least, signs of resisting examination. In patients under the age of 20, even those presenting soon after injury, the policy is more liberal and craniotomy is performed even if the highest response was no more than the ability to localize pain. Even with such apparently stringent criteria for operation, it has to be said that morbidity is still disappointingly high.

CEREBRAL OEDEMA

A rise in intracranial pressure that is not due to a localized collection of blood can occur after head injury as a result of brain swelling due to cerebral contusion, laceration, hypoxia, or ischaemia. In many rapidly fatal injuries, massive cerebral oedema occurs almost immediately after the impact and as a result of distension of the entire cerebral vascular bed, with vasoparalysis and failure of normal cerebral autoregulation. But there is no basis for the common assumption that unconsciousness after head injury is always accompanied by intracranial hypertension which demands the routine use of measures to reduce it. Some of the most deeply unconscious patients who survive in a persistent vegetative state have subatmospheric pressures from the earliest stages, unless of course they have been anoxic from respiratory obstruction. Cerebral oedema presents clinically with deteriorating consciousness, increase in focal neurological deficit or increase in restlessness, and it cannot be differentiated clearly from an acute surface haematoma, especially one in the subdural space. A swollen brain is also probable in those patients who are in a state of decerebrate rigidity almost from the moment of injury.

Raised intracranial pressure may be dealt with in different ways and using a variety of agents; they can conveniently be lumped together as 'brain shrinkers'. An indiscriminate reduction in pressure may mask a developing haematoma. As a general principle, therefore, 'brain shrinkers' should be used only in three situations:

1. When intracranial haematoma has been excluded.
2. To buy time for surgery when the decision to operate has already been made, but the patient is getting rapidly worse.
3. Where neurological deterioration is clearly related to an hypoxic episode before which the patient's level of consciousness had been high and stable.

The methods commonly employed fall into three main categories: pharmacological, mechanical and surgical.

Dehydration in some form or other is popular in the management of acute head injury. Most head injuries occur in previously healthy individuals in whom a few hours or even a day without fluids can do no harm, and after this time the vast majority have regained consciousness sufficiently to make up the deficit by mouth. Unless injury elsewhere calls for blood transfusion, an intravenous infusion need not be set up in the first instance. A hypertonic solution of magnesium sulphate given rectally is an old standby in neurosurgical practice; I have no personal experience of it, having always viewed the exercise with some distaste if only because it gives an already overworked nursing staff more to do than is necessary. Diuretics are much more convenient and act more quickly; the one of choice is Frusemide, in an adult dose of 20—40 mg either intravenously or by intramuscular injection. Hypertonic solutions given intravenously form the basis of most methods of reducing intracranial pressure, the main drawback being the rebound that occurs after an early lowering in pressure, with the risk that the final pressure reached may be even higher than the initial one. Arguments about the relative merits of the different solutions do not appear to have any convincing data to support them, and the impression is that the more quickly and effectively the solution acts, the greater the rebound. They all work by attracting extracellular fluid into the circulating blood, which consequently increases blood volume until the kidneys excrete the excess fluid; in theory at least, if the volume of blood circulating is increased in the critical period when cerebral autoregulation has failed and the cerebral resistance vessels are no longer able to function, the rise in systemic arterial pressure may be directly transmitted to the cerebral capillary bed, with a paradoxical rise in intracranial pressure. However, the rise in circulating blood volume can be offset in part by giving Frusemide i.v. at the start of the infusion.

Mannitol in a dose of 1.5 to 2g/Kg given over a period of 30-60 minutes in 20 per cent or 25 per cent solution is perhaps the most widely used agent. The solutions are supersaturated at the strengths recommended, the solubility of Mannitol being 17.5 per cent, and they tend to crystallize out in storage; the bottle needs to be warmed in a water-bath to 50—60°C to redissolve the crystals before use. In the hectic atmosphere of an accident room with a very ill patient, such measures are likely to be overlooked. A 15 per cent solution is safer, and a dose of 1g per Kg is probably adequate. If the intracranial pressure has risen to a stage where cerebral autoregulation is impaired, it tends to follow passively any changes in systemic arterial pressure; in such a circumstance, the increase in blood pressure produced by the infusion of a large volume of hypertonic solution may actually raise the intracranial pressure instead of reducing it as intended and thus harm the patient. Urea (dose 1—1.5g/Kg) is far more effective, but this solution too takes about 20 minutes to prepare; the dangers of extravasation into soft tissues are considerable and urea is not an ideal drug in inexperienced hands.

In all forms of dehydration therapy there should be a constant guard against the dangers of electrolyte imbalance. Also, I believe that the extensive use of dehydration increases the probability of ischaemic brain damage. Stagnation of blood is a feature common to vessels in all contused tissue, as is the tendency for red cells to sludge; dehydration increases the chances of thrombosis in such blood vessels.

Corticosteroids play a major part in the control of cerebral oedema associated with brain tumours; the most popular drug is dexamethasone in an initial dose of 10 mg intravenously, followed by 4—5 mg every six hours. Whether the dose is 4 or 5 mg is immaterial, practice being influenced by the relative strengths of the products marketed by two proprietary firms — one preparation contains 4 mg per ml and the other 5 mg. Betamethasone is equally effective, but has somehow not found widespread popularity, though in the United Kingdom its use would help to conserve valuable foreign exchange.

In patients with cerebral tumour, intracranial pressure monitoring indicates that corticosteroids rarely achieve much reduction in pressure in less than 24 hours. Nevertheless dramatic improvement in the clinical state is often seen much earlier. It is assumed that this improvement, which occurs before there has been a reduction in pressure, is due to an increased cerebral compliance; that is, at the same level of pressure the skull can accommodate a larger volume of contents without jeopardizing cerebral autoregulation. Unfortunately, what evidence there is suggests that corticosteroids are ineffective, even in very high dosage, in the reduction of intracranial pressure in patients with head injury (Gudeman, Miller and Becker, 1979). Yet their routine administration is widespread and is an example of how, once a treatment of hypothetical value has been taken up, it acquires respectability, becomes incorporated into standard protocols, and continues to be used even after it has been shown to have no merit.

Of all the methods of reducing intracranial pressure, the one most readily available and rapid in action is controlled ventilation. The contribution of this technique to the reduction in the morbidity of cranial surgery has been so profound that no neurosurgeon nowadays would even think of carrying out an operation without it. Despite its proven efficacy in elective procedures, respiratory treatment has not been as widely applied in the management of trauma as some ardent protagonists of the regimen would wish.

Mechanical Ventilation in the Management of Trauma

Hypoxia in subtle forms that cannot be corrected merely by attention to the airway or administration of oxygen-enriched air or tracheotomy is a major problem in all forms of severe trauma and needs the more flexible support that artificial ventilation provides. In the United Kingdom as a whole there has been no argument over the need to ventilate the patient with a flail chest, whether associated with head injury or not. Ross (1970) demonstrated the importance of hypoxia in producing the early neurological symptoms in fat embolism, without there necessarily being any accompanying cyanosis or obvious respiratory signs. He emphasized the value of blood gas analysis as an aid to diagnosis, with assisted ventilation as a natural corollary in its management. Even in the absence of either injury to the head and chest or fat embolism, major trauma is associated with pulmonary insufficiency. The literature dealing with the mechanisms of post-traumatic pulmonary dysfunction is voluminous but we seem to be no closer to a clear understanding of the problems of pathology, though we accept that intravascular coagulation following severe tissue damage is a factor of importance. The end result of the pulmonary changes is terminal airway closure with continued perfusion of blood through the alveoli, producing hypoxaemia. Clinical and experimental studies of blood gases after injury have shown that quite severe respiratory insufficiency can exist in the presence of visually adequate chest excursions and a satisfactory skin colour. Powers and his colleagues (1972) studied 36 consecutive patients admitted to a 'shock unit'. Twenty-three of them met the definition for massive injury, *viz.* a systolic blood pressure of 80 mmHg (10.6 kPa) or less, requiring at least three pints of blood, without injury to the head or thorax. Of these 23 patients, 12 developed the respiratory distress syndrome, with arterial PaO_2 of less than 8 kPa. They concluded that an arterial O_2 saturation of less than 10 kPa was an indication for ventilator treatment.

When head injury and shock due to systemic trauma occur together, as is all too common in high speed vehicle accidents, there is always a possibility of either hypoxic hypoxia from airway obstruction before rescue, or cerebral ischaemic hypoxia from shock. Acute brain swelling results if hypoxic hypoxia is followed by arterial hypertension, frequent in severe head injury, or when systemic arterial pressure is restored to normal after ischaemic cerebral hypoxia.

Controlled ventilation in such a situation, instituted at the same time as other resuscitative measures, would not only reduce brain swelling but also in theory improve blood flow through ischaemic areas of brain more readily than by any other means. Controlled hyperventilation produces constriction in the still reactive vessels in unaffected areas of the brain, leading to a decrease in intracranial blood volume and intracranial pressure. This in turn improves passively tissue perfusion pressure in the diseased areas of brain with impaired vasomotor responses, producing a shift of regional blood flow to them.

Even in head injuries of less severity, provided that there is some impairment of consciousness, the responsiveness of the cerebral blood flow to adverse alterations in arterial oxygen or pH is reduced and there is cerebral hypoxia, as judged by the PO_2 in the cerebrospinal fluid. Controlled ventilation has therefore a dual role in the management of severe head injury: both in the control of intracranial pressure and in the correction of cerebral hypoxia. Attempts to correct hypoxia in patients with very high intracranial pressure simply by increasing oxygen concentration in inspired air may even increase the degree of cerebral hypoxia. Moody, Ruamsuke and Mullan (1969) observed the changes that occur in respiration, in intracranial pressure and in blood gases when cerebral compression is induced experimentally in dogs: as pressure rises, early and progressive alterations occure in respiratory patterns and, in later stages, the sensitivity of central chemoreceptors to CO_2 and pH is depressed; the primary chemical drive becomes peripheral and hypoxic; giving oxygen without mechanical support deprives the animal of this only remaining respiratory drive.

In spite of all the theoretical evidence supporting the use of controlled ventilation in the early stages of head injury, there is considerable variation in the extent to which the technique is applied. Thus on the continent of Europe and in the United States there is a tendency to use it much more freely and aggressively than in the United Kingdom. Our reluctance probably stems in part from a fear that such intensive measures may save life at the expense of a persistent vegetative state. Furthermore, Newcastle experience has been that, in patients with head injury alone, moderate decrease in arterial oxygen concentration has not been associated with such worsening of prognosis as has been reported elsewhere. The question is a difficult one to resolve because most of the clinical criteria used in assessment of severity are obscured by the early institution of ventilation, so that comparison between ventilated and non-ventilated patients in a controlled experiment is unreliable.

In Newcastle our approach to controlled ventilation, except in chest injuries and fat embolism, has been as an adjunct to other methods of reducing intracranial pressure when the latter have proved ineffective. The occasional exception has been the hyperventilating, decerebrate patient under 21 years of age, with intact brain stem reflexes and hypertonic limbs and with an arterial PCO_2 of less than 3.3 kPa. This is a group that we believe to have a chance of survival, and controlled ventilation may be instituted in the hope of improving cerebral blood flow and reducing morbidity. The Belfast experience with bullet wounds of the brain, where hyperventilation has played a beneficial role in the reduction of both mortality and morbidity, seems conclusive. Fortunately we have had no opportunity to verify their results. We have specifically avoided ventilator support in severely head-injured patients who have developed apnoea before admission to the neurological centre, and who have total absence of response to pain, widely dilated nonreacting pupils and flaccidity of all limbs. In a patient who stops breathing on the threshold of the unit, ventilation is carried on until any incidental haematomas have been dealt with surgically; but it is not persevered with if spontaneous respiration does not return at the end of operation, and if it seems unlikely that the kidneys will be available for transplant. To continue artificial respiration till the circulation fails, which may take several days, is not necessarily kind to the relatives or a responsible use of scarce and expensive resources. Emotions generated on this score are better directed towards the prevention of brain injury than in futile gestures after the brain has died. If the inability to reduce intracranial hypertension by simpler methods is an indication for institution of controlled hyperventilation, it is important to define the ways in which such a decision may be reached. The judgement can only be made on the basis of continuous monitoring of intracranial pressures.

Intracranial Pressure Monitoring

Since Lundberg first published his monograph on the continuous recording of ventricular fluid pressure in 1960, measurement of intracranial pressure has become standard practice in many neurosurgical units. Price (1980) has reviewed the technical aspects of monitoring. Doubts have often been expressed about whether routine monitoring has added a further dimension to clinical judgement and has significantly influenced outcome. In the management of head injury, however, where there is no clear correlation between the clinical state and intracranial pressure, it is of crucial value to know its precise level and the effects of treatment upon it. Again, the extent to which such monitoring is used is dictated by individual circumstance. My personal practice is to monitor intracranial pressure continuously in that particular group of patients where neurological deterioration or decerebration has led, after localized masses have been excluded, to a diagnosis of brain swelling. Even where the former possibility has been ruled out by radiological investigation, it is advisable to confirm the actual presence of brain swelling with a single burr hole, preferably in the right frontal region, where an intraventricular catheter or appropriate miniature transducer may be inserted according to individual preference. There is no agreement about the relative merits of the various techniques used and their reliability. Because in practice one is not interested in absolute values so much as in the rate of change in pressure, arguments about whether pressures should be measured in the lateral ventricle, in the subdural space or extradurally are superfluous, and there is little to choose between the various techniques available. The writer has used a miniature transducer introduced subdurally in the early part of his experience, but since 1968 has preferred to place the same transducer extradurally.

The aim has been to start continuous monitoring as soon as a haematoma has been ruled out or treated and the presence of a tense swollen brain has been confirmed. Once the diagnosis is made, the patient is given dexamethasone 10 mg combined with Frusemide 40 mg intravenously and a 10 per cent glycerol infusion is started, 500 ml being given over at least a two-hour period. The glycerol is given more rapidly if a catheter has previously been introduced to measure central venous pressure, the speed of infusion being as high as possible without increasing central venous pressure. If intracranial pressure is greater than 40 (5.3 kPa) and is continuing to rise, or if it is more than 50 (6.7 kPa) when first measured, intermittent positive pressure ventilation is used till the pressure is lowered to below 30 (4 kPa). There is a tendency for patients, other than those who are deeply unconscious, to fight the respirator, and an injection of diazepam or pancuronium bromide may be required. Ventilation is adjusted to maintain the P_aCO_2 between 3.5 and 4 kPa and the P_aO_2 above 14 kPa, the main emphasis being on the P_aCO_2; but it is discontinued if no fall in pressure is achieved within two hours. Dexamethasone is continued at a dose of 5 mg six-hourly for at least five days. Frusemide 40 mg and glycerol 100 g daily are also given for at least the first two days. It is my impression, in spite of opinions to the contrary, that corticosteroids will act in those patients that have reacted satisfactorily to ventilation, but their action takes at least 24 hours. Because of reservations about intensive dehydration, even with careful attention to serum electrolytes and fluid balance, we prefer to discontinue diuretics and hypertonic solutions after 48 hours.

Unfortunately, not all patients in whom intracranial pressure monitoring is desirable are suitable for the procedure. A number, for whom knowledge of the rate of change of pressure would be most valuable and whose response to treatment might be anticipated, are so restless and unco-operative that monitoring is not feasible. Furthermore, there is a natural reluctance to expose expensive apparatus to the risk of damage. Patients with temporal lobe contusion are among those in whom such problems arise; most of them are treated conservatively with dehydration and steroids alone, and few need lobectomy. Because of their level of consciousness they often will not tolerate an indwelling monitor without tugging at it, and it becomes necessary to fall back on clinical judgement to assess the efficacy of treatment. However, monitoring is undoubtedly the ideal to be aimed at, for it enables us to assess progress and at the same time to anticipate clinical deterioration; for instance, the appearance of plateau waves (that is, sustained rises of intracranial pressure approaching diastolic blood pressure) provides advance warning of a change for the worse in a patient's condition. However, temporal lobe contusions, though in my experience as frequent as subacute subdural haematomas, have not been a particular problem in management; nor has that other fortunately rare group suffering from the so-called 'talk and die' syndrome, all of whom do *not* die if treated adequately and early.

'Lucid' Interval Without Haematoma

Most patients who, having spoken after injury, later become unconscious, harbour an intracranial haematoma — either subdural or extradural. No standard textbook of surgery even refers to the possibility of such deterioration in the absence of haematoma, and yet it is a situation that does arise and is sometimes fatal. In most instances the deterioration can be explained on the basis of hypoxia, but there still remains a very small separate group with a distinctive clinical pattern. When first seen in the casualty department, the patient is able to give his name and sometimes his address, but he is restless even to the point of being violent, unco-operative and abusive. Should his breath smell of alcohol, his state is naturally ascribed to this in most cases correctly. If one can get near enough to examine him, the external point of impact is usually seen to be at the back of the head; he has photophobia and meningism. This general state is one which the older textbooks called 'cerebral irritation'. Though talking, he is never actually lucid. He looks at first as if he should recover in a few hours once the effects of the alcohol have worn off. However, there is increasing restlessness, sometimes so difficult to control that in the interests of other patients in the ward he is sedated. The subsequent deterioration to coma that may thereby be accelerated is, not unnaturally, at first attributed only to the sedation. Should the progressive increase in restlessness lead to angiography because of suspicion of haematoma, the appearances are likely to be those of intense and widespread arterial spasm, with or without midline displacement and a slow cerebral circulation. If an exploratory burr hole is made, the brain is likely to be soft and tense; it may herniate through the dural incision in the manner of toothpaste. It it were possible to monitor the patient's intracranial pressure at the stage of restlessness, it would be easier to judge the effects of attempted therapy. As it is, treatment tends to be empirical and to depend on diuretics, hypertonic solutions and dexamethasone. As the clinical and radiological features point to ischaemic brain injury from traumatic subarachnoid haemorrhage and arterial spasm, it seems inappropriate to apply energetic dehydration; at the same time it is difficult in so rare a condition to build up sufficient experience to determine whether hyperventilation or surgical decompression by extensive bifrontal craniotomy has any advantages over simpler pharmacological methods of reducing pressure. All three methods at one time or another have ended in death or a persistent vegetative state. No patient who has become deeply unconscious and unable to localize pain in this condition has made a worthwhile recovery and, in the absence of information derived from pressure recording, it is difficult to assess the part that treatment has played in cases of lesser severity where recovery has taken place.

Hypothermia and Hyperbaric Oxygen

These certainly deserve mention in a discussion of methods of reducing intracranial pressure and improving cerebral blood flow. Lowering body temperature to 30°C reduces cerebral metabolism by about 30 per cent and it also reduces brain tension. However, it is an inconvenient procedure, with a number of technical drawbacks, and stable temperatures are difficult to maintain in an unanaesthetized patient. There is a tendency for the temperature to drift downwards, with consequent danger of cardiac irregularity and arrest. In general the technique seems to be less popular than it was at one time; in Newcastle its use is limited to the reduction of hyperpyrexia. We have no experience of hyperbaric oxygen in neurosurgical practice; it has been shown to be effective experimentally but there is no evidence that its use is in any way superior to controlled ventilation, which is so much more readily available.

SKULL FRACTURE

For most laymen, skull fracture has sinister connotations. Not infrequently a relative of a deeply unconscious patient will enquire whether or not there is skull fracture, and the information that there is not seems to afford a quite unwarrantable sense of relief which is undiminished by the obviously critical appearance of the patient. A skull fracture on its own without injury to associated structures does not affect the outcome of head injury. The question of surgery arises in depressed and compound fractures of the skull. There is never any need for an emergency operation, unless of course there is evidence of an associated haematoma with cerebral compression. The timing and type of operation are governed by the nature and situation of the fracture. Management may be considered under three headings: simple depressed fracture, compound fracture of the vault and compound fracture of the skull base.

Simple Depressed Fracture

The usual practice is to elevate fractures in which the depression is greater than the thickness of the vault. There is, however, no evidence that the advantages are any more than cosmetic or psychological. It seems unlikely that the chances of post-traumatic epilepsy will be reduced, as is often supposed, because the damage will have been done already. An obvious palpable depression, even when covered by hair, may become the focus of attention in a patient with a disability resulting from brain injury. The patient or his relatives may blame persistence of the disability on the fact that an operation was not undertaken to raise the fracture. The decision whether or not to operate may therefore be quite a complex one and it may to some extent depend on the attitudes of patients or relatives. There is no doubt that any cranial operation, however trivial, increases the chance of psychological morbidity and induces the impression in the lay mind that the injury was of greater severity than it might have been. Operation for depressed fracture can in fact be deferred for several days so that all the various factors may be taken into account.

Compound Fracture of Skull Vault

A compound fracture of the vault of the skull is probably the most likely kind to be missed. There may be no history of concussion and x-ray of skull may be omitted or possibly misinterpreted. The basic principles governing management are those that apply to compound fractures elsewhere in the body: exploration of the wound to remove contaminated and nonviable tissue, followed by primary closure to prevent infection. If the dura underneath the fracture is not lacerated, the risk of neglect is, at most, that of osteomyelitis; but where the dura has been penetrated, meningitis and cerebral abscess are much more hazardous prospects. It is not always possible to assess the exact state of affairs under the fracture either clinically or radiologically and the operation must therefore be regarded as exploratory. It need not be carried out immediately after injury and in cases of multiple trauma it is reasonable to delay operation for a few hours until it becomes clear that no remote complications, such as ruptured spleen, are developing. With the use of antibiotics, to delay surgery for up to 24 hours does not in any way influence the morbidity.

In the relatively straight forward situation of a scalp laceration over a linear undepressed fracture, no more is required than careful cleaning of the laceration and closure, along with antibiotics for two weeks. The author has a preference for penicillin and sulphadimidine rather than broad spectrum antibiotics, on the assumption that the patient newly arrived in hospital is unlikely to be carrying the resistant organisms that the indiscriminate use of antibiotics has created in the hospital environment. Bearing in mind the mechanism of fracture, in that bone is driven in at the point of impact, a case could be made for routine exploration of the dura under the fracture line. Indeed there are undoubtedly instances where patients operated on for reasons such as haematoma are found to have dural lacerations, which would not otherwise have been discovered, directly under an undepressed fracture. In such circumstances even linear lacerations of the cortex may be encountered unexpectedly. In compound depressed fractures, the inner table is generally damaged over a greater area than the outer; the fragments are often impacted and there is more to the operation than simply the elevation of depressed bone. Therefore an adequate exposure is essential, either by enlarging the original laceration or, if the latter is small, by turning a scalp flap after suturing the laceration. If the dura is intact, it is safer not to open it unless there is suspicion of underlying haematoma, in which case the dura is blue in colour and does not pulsate. If the dura is torn, the search for indriven foreign bodies will necessitate opening it up more widely, and small intradural haematomas may be found. Softened necrotic brain tissue is removed by gentle suction to leave a clean bed of normal-looking brain which is not under tension. The dura should always be repaired. If a free graft is needed it is obtained from the adjacent pericranium or temporal fascia, although large wounds may necessitate taking a piece of fascia lata from the thigh. If there are bone fragments that are not too contaminated or comminuted, they are washed in saline and replaced. This is particularly desirable in children. A primary repair of a skull defect with an inert prosthesis may be carried out if bone fragments are too small to be replaced; such a step spares the patient a second operation for cosmetic repair at a later date. Acrylic is most readily available and it can be moulded on the spot. In children a tantalum plate, again highly malleable, can be shaped to the skull contour and sutured to the pericranium with silk sutures. I have not used tantalum for primary repair because of an aversion to allowing metal to come into contact with denuded bone; this is combined with a reluctance to wire the plate to bone because the only cases of wound infection from tantalum plates have been when the plate has been screwed into the bone, or fastened with wire passing through holes drilled in the bone. One of the most important aims of cranial surgery is the prevention of infection and, if there is doubt about bone fragments, they are better discarded and cranioplasty postponed until a later date.

The high incidence of late complications from neglected or missed compound depressed fractures discourages a conservative approach in the management of a small group where surgery itself may contribute to morbidity. This would apply to depressed compound fractures with clean small lacerations over them, especially if they lie over a major dural venous sinus. The unfortunate complications that do occur are, for instance, where the patient has not bothered to report an apparently trivial head wound, or where antibiotics have not been given after the suture of a scalp laceration in a patient who has not undergone skull x-ray.

Missile injuries fall into a special group. The velocity of impact will determine the extent to which tissue is disrupted and management may call for more complex measures than the straightforward surgery referred to so far. In the absence of personal experience, one may turn to the unique work from Belfast (Gordon, 1975). Generally, after injury the clinical state is labile, shock and blood loss may be severe, and deterioration in consciousness ending in death may occur in spite of prompt resuscitation, controlled ventilation and early though not immediate surgery (Crockard, 1974). In the Belfast study, patients with uncontrollable haemorrhage or signs of an expanding haematoma were operated on immediately, but otherwise hyperventilation was continued for at least an hour before operation. Surgery consisted of extensive debridement, careful haemostasis, dural closure usually with a fascial graft and, in many cases, rotation scalp flaps with appropriate skin grafting. Although bone fragments were generally removed, metallic fragments were found to penetrate much deeper, and fewer than half the bullets were retrieved. The level of consciousness on admission was a direct influence on outcome. Crockard found that the mortality was 11.5 per cent in those who were initially alert, rose to 33.3 per cent if the patient was drowsy, and to 79.1 per cent if reacting to pain only, while no patient in coma survived. The deterioration was usually due to cerebral oedema; hyperventilation was continued after operation for as long as necessary, but only if there was apparent improvement on clinical assessment for which the patient was decurarized at intervals of 24—48 hours. Primary skull repair was not carried out.

Compound Fracture of the Base of the Skull

As in the previous section, surgery for fractures of the base of the skull is essentially prophylactic to prevent intracranial infection. The indications for surgery are somewhat controversial, and individual surgeons may be inconsistent in their approach. Thus a surgeon who is inclined towards a radical approach may advocate exploration of all patients with c.s.f. rhinorrhoea, and yet adopt a different attitude to c.s.f. otorrhoea. A decision to operate may of course be influenced by the situation of a probable fistula. Thus a fracture of the clivus opening into a large sphenoid air sinus might pose a problem in a young patient. In years gone by there were considerable problems of access, but nowadays the opening can be plugged through a trans-sphenoidal approach. In elderly and debilitated patients there is some hesitation about embarking on such operations.

There is little argument about the need to operate where rhinorrhoea or otorrhoea is persistent or profuse, or if the patient has had an attack of meningitis. Where rhinorrhoea has been transient, surgery is advised if x-rays of the skull show more than a hairline fracture, because cessation of c.s.f. discharge may be due to the fact that the dural defect has been occluded by a small cerebral fungus. Surgery is also indicated in cases with transient rhinorrhoea without fracture who have bilateral anosmia.

Where an aerocoele is seen on x-ray in patients without rhinorrhoea, operation is advised if the air does not show signs of absorption within a few days. It has not been our policy to operate on patients with fractures through the paranasal sinuses even in the absence of rhinorrhoea, aerocoele or an opaque sinus on x-ray, as is advocated by some authors. The indications are not influenced by the presence of faciomaxillary fractures; in two-thirds of patients with such fractures, c.s.f. rhinorrhoea for some of the time was observed by Leopard (1970) in his review of 116 cases. When a patient is first admitted to hospital, prophylactic penicillin and sulphadimidine are started if there are any clinical signs of a fracture of the base, even if there is no rhinorrhoea or aerocoele. Where either is present, the patient is advised not to blow his nose. Lumbar drainage of c.s.f. in an effort to reduce the rhinorrhoea is not practice, as the lowering of pressure may increase risks of meningitis. In c.s.f. otorrhoea, no action is taken beyond prophylactic antibiotics and a gauze pad over the ear to catch drips on to the pillow. In all cases antibiotics are continued for at least a fortnight after the c.s.f. leak has clearly stopped.

Operation is never carried out as an emergency; the morbidity is much less if it is delayed till the patient has recovered fully from any post-traumatic brain swelling, the best external sign being disappearance of scalp bruising and oedema, usually after the tenth day. If the patient has already developed meningitis, this is treated before operation is considered. Because most dural tears in the anterior cranial fossa are very close to the midline and may cross it, a bifrontal craniotomy is generally used and both sides explored. Repair is as a rule much easier in otorrhoea, though less often required, as the fistula is almost always quite superficial on the tegmen tympani.

PROBLEMS OF PROLONGED UNCONSCIOUSNESS

In the prevention of respiratory complications, tracheostomy need not be carried out at a very early stage, as endotracheal intubation can be continued for a week or more without difficulty. By this time a clearer idea of the prognosis may have emerged. Tracheostomy is certainly not recommended in elderly patients with severe head injuries or in younger patients with flaccid limbs and absence of pupillary and corneal reflexes. In cases of less severe injury the presence of facial fracture, chest damage, injury to spine or extremities requiring prolonged immobilization in the supine position — all these may be indications for tracheostomy. It is doubtful, however, that the operation has anything to offer in patients with a good cough reflex; even the most skilled nursing care of the tracheostomy cannot clear the smallest bronchioles as effectively as can the expulsive force of a cough when the back of the pharynx is stimulated by the introduction of a suction catheter. A tracheostomy deprives the patient of this important process.

Patients who are deeply unconscious after admission will, in most cases, have had a wide-bore nasogastric tube introduced to empty the stomach and keep it clear. If the patient has not recovered and is unable to swallow after 12 hours or so increasing volumes of fluid, starting with 30 ml water hourly, are given through the tube, if there is no aspirate. The feed is gradually increased in volume if the patient tolerates it, and is built up as rapidly as possible till it provides the daily nutritional intake in a total volume of two to 2.5 litres. Intravenous feeding is used only to make up quantities where the stomach cannot cope. The importance of careful attention to fluid balance, especially where there may be diabetes insipidus, should not be underestimated.

Space does not allow detailed consideration of the finer aspects of metabolic care. In many severe head injuries, the catabolic phase is prolonged well beyond the few days usual in severe trauma elsewhere; this is probably due to hypothalamic disturbance. We are not convinced that the parenteral administration of solutions containing a high concentration of amino acids has in any way reduced the almost relentless wasting that occurs.

DRUG THERAPY

The use of drugs for the treatment of brain swelling has already been dealt with. Otherwise the only drugs commonly used in the management of head injuries are antibiotics, either for respiratory complications or where compound fracture is suspected.

Even in the groups which are statistically most like to develop epilepsy, anti-convulsants are not given from the beginning as adequate serum levels are unlikely to be attained. In the occasional case of status epilepticus, phenytoin sodium and phenobarbitone sodium are started, the status being controlled either with intravenous diazepam or Amytal, for which I have a preference.

There is uncertainty about the practical value of giving routine anticonvulsants to patients who have had either an intracranial haematoma, a single convulsion in the first week, or dural penetration from a depressed fracture. Despite the experimental evidence in support of the prophylactic value of anticonvulsants in suppressing the formation of an epileptic focus, if these drugs are prescribed there is a great tendency for the patient to forget or fail to take them. This pattern is perhaps in keeping with the personality and temperament of a proportion of individuals who are prone to head injury.

Diabetes insipidus, when it occurs, is controlled with Pitressin by injection, or with desmopressin. Patients with decerebrate rigidity have been treated with regular doses of 'lytic cocktail' (i.e., chlorpromazine, promethazine and pethidine hydrochloride), 25 mg each i.v., to control both frequent decerebrate spasms and hyperpyrexia, if it accompanies them. In general, however, they are probably better treated by means of controlled ventilation.

CONCLUSION

It was not the intention in this chapter to cover all the problems that arise in the management of head injuries so much as to indicate some of the essentially unresolved aspects and to stimulate a reappraisal of long established notions. The views expressed reflect a personal experience that has to some extent modified the conventional learning with which I set out to deal with head injuries some 20 years ago. No attempt has been made at completeness; for instance, it has not seemed appropriate to include consideration of some of the rarer surgical problems, such as caroticocavernous fistula and occult hydrocephalus.

REFERENCES

Ambrose, J., Gooding, M. R. & Uttley, D. (1976) EMI scan in the management of injuries. *Lancet,* i, 847-848.
Becker, D. P., Miller, J. D., Ward, D. D., Greenberg, R. P., Young, H. F. & Sakalas, R. (1977) The outcome from severe head injury with early diagnosis and intensive treatment. *Journal of Neurosurgery,* 47, 491-502.
Cairns, H. (1941) Rehabilitation after injuries to the central nervous system. *Proceedings of the Royal Society of Medicine,* 35, 299-302.
Crockard, H. A. (1974) Bullet injuries of the brain. *Annals of the Royal College of Surgeons, England,* 55, 111-123.
French, B. N. & Dublin, B. (1977) The value of computerized tomography in the management of 1000 consecutive head injuries. *Surgical Neurology,* 7, 171-183.
Galbraith, S. L. (1973) Age distribution of extradural haemorrhage without skull fracture. *Lancet,* i, 1217-1218.
Gallagher, J. P. & Browder, E. J. (1968) Extradural haematoma; experience with 167 patients. *Journal of Neurosurgery,* 29, 1-12.
Gordon, D. S. (1975) Missile wounds of the head and spine. *British Medical Journal,* i, 614-616.
Gudeman, S. K., Miller, J. D. & Becker, D. P. (1979) Failure of high-dosage steroid therapy to influence intracranial pressure in patients with severe head injury. *Journal of Neurosurgery,* 51, 301-306.
Harwood-Nash, D. C., Hendrick, E. B. & Hudson, A. R. (1971) The significance of skull fractures in children. A study of 1187 patients. *Paediatric Radiology,* 101, 151-155.
Hooper, R. (1969) *Patterns of Acute Head Injury,* pp. 54-63. London: Edward Arnold.
Jamieson, K. G. (1970) Extradural and subdural haematomas. Changing patterns and requirements of treatment in Australia. *Journal of Neurosurgery,* 33, 632-635.

Jamieson, K. G. & Yelland, J. D. N. (1968) Extradural haematoma: 167 cases. *Journal of Neurosurgery,* **29,** 13-23.

Jennett, B., Teasdale, G., Galbraith, S., Pickard, J., Grant, H., Braakman, R., Avezaat, C., Maas, A., Minderhoud, J., Vecht, C. J., Heiden, J., Small, R., Caton, W. & Kurze, T. (1977) Severe head injuries in three countries. *Journal of Neurology, Neurosurgery and Psychiatry,* **40,** 291-298.

Jennett, B., Teasdale, G., Fry, J., Braakman, R., Minderhoud, J., Heiden, J. & Kurze, T. (1980) Treatment for severe head injury. *Journal of Neurology, Neurosurgery and Psychiatry,* **43,** 289-295.

Leopard, P. (1970) Dural tears in maxillo-facial injuries. *British Journal of Oral Surgery,* **8,** 222-230.

Lundberg, N. (1960) Continuous recording and control of ventricular fluid pressure in neurosurgical practice. *Acta Psychiatrica Scandinavica* (Supplement) **149.**

McIver, I. N., Lassman, L. P., Thomson, C. W. & McLeod, I. (1958) Treatment of severe head injuries. *Lancet,* **ii,** 544-550.

Moody, R. A., Ruamsuke, S. & Mullan, S. F. (1969) Experimental effects of acutely increased intracranial pressure on respiration and blood gases. *Journal of Neurosurgery,* **30,** 482-493.

Powers, S. R. Jr., Burdge, R., Leather, R., Monaco, V., Newell, J., Sardar, S. & Smith, E. J. (1972) Studies of pulmonary insufficiency in non-thoracic trauma. *Journal of Trauma,* **12,** 1-14.

Price, D. J. E. (1980) Intracranial pressure monitoring. *British Journal of Clinical Equipment,* **5,** 92-98.

Price, D. J. E. & Murray, A. (1972) The influence of hypoxia and hypotension on recovery from head injury. *Injury,* **3,** 218-224.

Relander, M., Troupp, H. & Bjorkesten, G. (1972) Controlled trial of treatment for cerebral concussion. *British Medical Journal,* **iv,** 777-779.

Ross, A. P. J. (1970) The fat embolism syndrome with special reference to the importance of hypoxia in the syndrome. *Annals of the Royal College of Surgeons, England,* **46,** 159-171.

Sevitt, S. (1968) Fatal road accidents, injuries, complications and causes of death in 250 subjects. *British Journal of Surgery,* **55,** 481-505.

Teasdale, G. & Jennett, W. B. (1974) Assessment of coma and impaired consciousness — a practical scale. *Lancet,* **ii,** 81-84.

Thomson, C. & Longley, B. P. (1965) (Personal communication).

Tindall, G. T., Patton, J. M., Dunion, J. J. & O'Brien, M. S. (1975) Monitoring of patients with head injuries. *Clinical Neurosurgery,* **22,** 332-363.

Walker, A. E. (1966) Introduction, Chapter 1. In *Head Injury: Conference Proceedings* (Ed.) Caveness, W. F. & Walker, A. E., p. 22. Philadelphia: J. B. Lippincott.

Wood Jones, F. (1912) The vascular lesion in some cases of middle meningeal haemorrhage, *Lancet,* **ii,** 7-12.

Index

199